Prehospital Care of Neurologic Emergencies

Edited by

Todd J. Crocco, MD
Professor and Chair, Department of Emergency Medicine,
West Virginia University School of Medicine,
Morgantown, WV, USA

Michael R. Sayre, MD
Professor, Division of Emergency Medicine,
University of Washington, Seattle, WA, USA

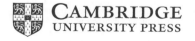

CAMBRIDGE
UNIVERSITY PRESS

CAMBRIDGE
UNIVERSITY PRESS

University Printing House, Cambridge CB2 8BS, United Kingdom

Cambridge University Press is part of the University of Cambridge.

It furthers the University's mission by disseminating knowledge in the pursuit of education, learning and research at the highest international levels of excellence.

www.cambridge.org
Information on this title: www.cambridge.org/9781107678323

© Cambridge University Press 2014

First published 2014

Printed in the United Kingdom by Clays, St Ives plc

A catalogue record for this publication is available from the British Library

Library of Congress Cataloguing in Publication data
Prehospital care of neurologic emergencies / edited by Todd J. Crocco, Michael R. Sayre.
   p. ; cm.
Includes bibliographical references and index.
ISBN 978-1-107-67832-3 (Paperback)
I. Crocco, Todd, editor of compilation.   II. Sayre, Michael, editor of compilation.
[DNLM: 1. Nervous System Diseases.   2. Emergency Medical Services. WL 140]
RC350.N49
616.8'0425–dc23   2014000265

ISBN 978-1-107-67832-3 Paperback

....

To my wife, Diane, who is the strongest and most understanding person I know and without whom my life would be empty – thank you for coming into my life and for every day we have together. To my daughters, Miranda and Morgan, who are a never-ending source of pride and joy in my life. I love you all more than my words can ever express. – Todd J. Crocco

To my wife, Diana, who provides limitless encouragement, I love you and hope you will continue to press me to enjoy life. To my children, Eric, Allison and Kevin: May you strive to excel in love and remember to Pay Forward. – Michael R. Sayre

TABLE OF CONTENTS

CONTRIBUTORS

Jane H. Brice, MD, MPH
Professor of Emergency Medicine, University of North
Carolina, Chapel Hill, NC, USA

Stephanie A. Crapo, MD
Department of Emergency Medicine, University of
North Carolina, Chapel Hill, NC, USA

J. Stephen Huff, MD
Professor of Emergency Medicine and Neurology,
University of Virginia, Charlottesville, VA, USA

Eric Jaeger, JD, NREMT-P
Paramedic, Lecturer and Consultant, True North Group,
NH, USA

Jeffrey Kelly, MS, NREMT-P
Maryland State Police – Aviation Command, Maryland
Institute for Emergency Medical Services Systems, MD, USA

Hollynn Larrabee, MD
Associate Professor of Emergency Medicine, West Virginia
University, Morgantown, WV, USA

Michael G. Millin, MD, MPH
Assistant Professor of Emergency Medicine, Johns Hopkins
University School of Medicine, Maryland Institute for
Emergency Medical Services Systems, MD, USA

Gregory P. Schaefer, DO
Assistant Professor of Surgery, West Virginia University,
Morgantown, WV, USA

Robert Silbergleit, MD
Professor of Emergency Medicine, University of Michigan,
Ann Arbor, MI, USA

Terry A. Taylor, II, EMT-P
Firefighter/Paramedic, EMSPlumbline, LLC, USA

Richard B. Utarnachitt, MD
Acting Assistant Professor of Emergency Medicine, University
of Washington, School of Medicine, Seattle, WA, USA

M. Kay Vonderschmidt, MPA, MS, NREMT-P
Department of Emergency Medicine, University of Cincinnati,
College of Medicine, Cincinnati, OH, USA

Leslie A. Willard, RN, CFRN
WVU Hospital and HealthNet Aeromedical Services,
Morgantown, WV, USA

John M. Wooten, BA, EMT-P
Orange County Emergency Services, Hillsborough, NC, USA

PREFACE

Real-life heroes do exist. They frequently emerge at times when we least expect it. Even though they rarely draw attention to themselves, they are not that hard to find. Consider, for example, the men and women who respond to the call for help every day in this country. It happens thousands of times every day. It's even happening right now.

In a moment of need, people often summon emergency medical service professionals for help. Their assistance can be required across the full spectrum of healthcare. From trauma to psychiatric emergencies, from cardiac to pediatric complaints, emergency medical service (EMS) providers need to be ready for anything. Owing to this lofty expectation, these healthcare providers are expected to have a wide breadth of knowledge and understanding. Invariably, there are certain types of emergencies that cause more alarm and anxiety even for the most experienced providers.

In our experience, neurologic emergencies are among the most challenging emergencies to manage in the back of an ambulance. Providing emergency personnel with the necessary advice and direction for complex neurologic emergencies will invariably be a welcomed relief for many. This book aims to provide just that. Designed to be succinct yet comprehensive enough to explain the basis for the recommendations, this book is intended to provide emergency caregivers with the answers they need on short notice when caring for a neurologic emergency.

The evidence presented in each chapter has been broken down into three levels of evidence:

- high-quality evidence – consistent evidence from randomized trials, or overwhelming evidence of some other form;
- moderate-quality evidence – evidence from randomized trials with important limitations, or very strong evidence of some other form;
- low-quality evidence – evidence from observational studies, unsystematic clinical observations, or from randomized trials with serious flaws.

It is our sincere hope that providing guidelines through this focused approach will be a useful aid in the prehospital management of neurologic emergencies for healthcare personnel at all levels.

Chapter 1

Lightheadedness and dizziness

Richard B. Utarnachitt

Recommendations

High quality

There are insufficient data to support a Level I
recommendation for this topic.

Moderate quality

The prehospital professional needs to determine which
patients presenting with a chief complaint of lightheadedness
or dizziness require emergent transport to a healthcare facility
for evaluation.

1. perform a blood sugar check;
2. obtain a 12 lead ECG;
3. complete a focused neurologic assessment (using
   prehospital stroke scales);
4. complete a focused cardiovascular assessment, including
   blood pressure readings from both arms.

Prehospital Care of Neurologic Emergencies, ed. Todd J. Crocco
and Michael R. Sayre. Published by Cambridge University Press.
© Cambridge University Press 2014.

Low quality

Detailed neurologic tests have been developed to rapidly assess a dizzy patient to determine if their symptoms are due to a benign versus malignant cause.

1. systolic blood pressure < 160 mmHg;
2. lack of horizontal nystagmus.[1]

Orthostatic vital signs are often used to determine if a patient is volume depleted. Although still taught as part of the evaluation of a dizzy patient, low-quality evidence suggests that the clinical value is limited.

Overview

A chief complaint of feeling "lightheaded or dizzy" is extremely common. The National Institutes of Health estimates that approximately 40 percent of all Americans will seek treatment for dizziness at some point in their lives.[2] This is especially true in the elderly population, who constitute the majority of patients with this complaint. Despite the relative frequency of patients presenting with a complaint of dizziness, studies directly addressing this population are quite sparse.

Most causes of dizziness are indeed benign. Common culprits include vestibular disorders such as benign peripheral positional vertigo or labyrinthitis, medication side effects and psychogenic causes. Although these are benign conditions, they can be so concerning and troublesome for the patient that EMS is activated when they occur. Conversely, there are more serious conditions that can present as dizziness. These include acute ischemic or hemorrhagic stroke, cerebral posterior circulation ischemia, cardiac dysrhythmias and acute dissection (aortic and carotid). Other systemic causes may also present as lightheadedness, such as acute myocardial infarction or sepsis. The prehospital professional must safely determine which patients require emergent diagnostic evaluation and intervention.

Physiology

In order to successfully approach patients who are complaining of dizziness, the EMS professional needs to understand how the brain perceives orientation in space and processes the signals to maintain an upright posture. Balance is a complex interplay between the vestibular organs of the peripheral system contained in the inner ear and the central vestibular system in the brain made up of the vestibular nuclei, cerebellum, brainstem, spinal cord and the vestibular cortex. The cerebellum plays a key role in the fine-tuning of this information. Any derangement in this pathway can be perceived as dizziness.[3]

The vestibular organs are housed within the bony labyrinth of the ear. This consists of the bony semicircular canals (superior, posterior and horizontal) and the vestibule (Figure 1.1). The membranous labyrinth fills the bony labyrinth consisting of the semicircular canals and the otolithic organs, the utricle and saccule, are within the vestibule. These semicircular canals are involved in sensing angular rotation. Each semicircular canal is positioned perpendicular from the

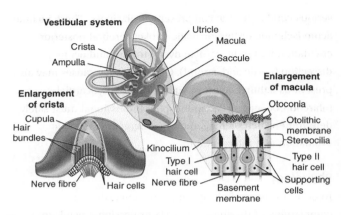

Figure 1.1 Anatomy of the inner ear. Adapted from reference Vestibular System (2013)[4]

other such that every possible rotational direction of movement can be sensed, i.e. in the X, Y and Z axes.

Within each canal is a fluid called endolymph. Movement of this fluid occurs based on the direction of rotation of the patient's head. This movement is subsequently sensed by a structure at the ends of each semicircular canal called the ampulla.

The ampulla houses the cupula, where hair-like structures called stereocilia project. Adjacent to each bunch of stereocilia is a single longer structure called the kinocilia that is the sensory portion of the structure. The kinocilia transmit a baseline signal to the vestibular nuclei even when stationary. During head rotation, endolymph movement in the semicircular canal is sensed in the corresponding cupula.

The stereocilia will either bend toward the sensing kinocilia causing increased frequency of discharges that will be sensed by the vestibular nuclei; or, conversely, the corresponding semicircular canal on the opposite side will bend away from the kinocilia, producing a diminished signal transmission indicating head turning in the opposite direction (Figure 1.1).

The otolithic organs (utricle and saccule) work on a similar premise as the semicircular canals. However, instead of angular rotation, they sense linear acceleration. The utricle senses linear movement in the horizontal plane, whereas the saccule senses upward and downward directions. As their name suggests, these organs also differ from the semicircular canals in that they contain otoconia, calcium carbonate stones which aid in the sensing of movement by providing inertia by the virtue of their increased mass. The hair cells and kinocilia in the utricle and saccule are imbedded in the otolithic membrane and are topped with otoconia. As movement occurs, the inertia imparted by the otoconia move the otolithic membrane either toward the sensing kinocilia, indicating the direction of movement, or away, indicating the opposite direction of movement (Figure 1.2).

Categories of dizziness

It is important to define what is meant by "dizziness." Traditionally, dizziness is often subdivided into four different categories: lightheadedness, presyncope, disequilibrium and vertigo.

"Lightheadedness" or non-specific dizziness is the most nebulous category and likely to be the most common of the

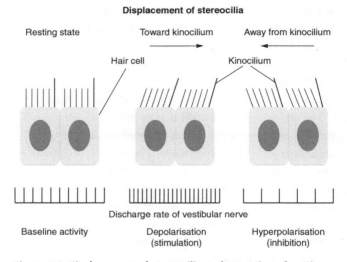

Figure 1.2 Displacement of stereocilia and sensation of motion. Reproduced with permission from reference Lee (2012)[3]

four complaints. Other descriptors associated with lightheadedness are terms like "wooziness" or "disconnected from body." A history of trauma as well as ingestion of vasoactive medications (anti-hypertensive drugs or rate-controlling agents) and psychiatric medications such as anti-psychotics or tricyclic anti-depressants may precede the symptoms. Psychogenic causes are more likely to be the culprit if the symptoms are prolonged, in excess of several months.[3, 5] The majority of patients with a complaint of lightheadedness do not need immediate intervention.

Presyncope is defined as a sensation of impending loss of consciousness. Presyncope may progress to syncope, which is a sudden and brief loss of consciousness as a result of global cerebral hypoperfusion.[5] Some patients complaining of presyncope have cardiac rhythm disturbances (e.g. too fast or too slow). Obtaining a 12 lead ECG may be helpful to determine if a cardiac dysrhythmia is the culprit. Other patients are excessively vasodilated and develop low mean arterial pressures. Some of these patients are taking antihypertensive medications or rate-control agents. Increased parasympathetic tone from activation of the vagus nerve slows heart rate and may lead to hypotension and then transient cerebral hypoperfusion. Symptoms should resolve if the patient is supine and worsen while sitting up or standing. Cardiac monitoring may identify profound bradycardia.

Vertigo is a sensation of false movement. The main challenge in evaluating a vertiginous patient is determining whether the problem is with the peripheral vestibular system versus central nervous system.

Peripheral causes involve the vestibular organs (described earlier). Problems arise when the peripheral vestibular structures (semicircular canals, utricle or saccule) sense movement when in fact there is none. This may occur due to inflammation or irritation of these structures. This disagreement between the two ears of the vestibular system and other balance-sensing mechanisms (visual system and somatosensory) gives rise to the sensation of vertigo. Etiologies for peripheral vertigo are not life-threatening. Common disorders include benign positional peripheral vertigo (BPPV), vestibular neuritis and labyrinthitis. Another term to describe these conditions is acute peripheral vestibulopathy (APV).[6]

Viral syndromes, local inflammation and medication side effects are the culprits in the vast majority of cases.

Central vertigo occurs when the portions of the central nervous system involved in balance, namely vestibular nuclei on the brain stem, vestibular cortex, spinal cord or the cerebellum, are injured or dead. Central causes of vertigo, unlike peripheral causes of vertigo, are often due to life-threatening conditions such as vertebrobasilar strokes, ischemia in the distribution of the posterior cerebral fossa, central nervous system (CNS) tumors, CNS infection, brain trauma or multiple sclerosis.[6, 7]

Disequilibrium is defined as a feeling of imbalance. This is not associated with a sense of false movement. Patients with disequilibrium will have difficulty ambulating and will often present with a wide, unsteady gait.[3] Causes of disequilibrium include peripheral neuropathy and musculoskeletal disorders.

Dizziness can be further subdivided into orthostatic dizziness and positional dizziness. Orthostatic dizziness implies symptoms that develop when the patient changes position in the vertical plane, i.e. from a position of supine or sitting to standing. Positional orthostasis refers to symptoms that develop when head position is changed. The presence of orthostatic dizziness implies autonomic dysfunction or volume depletion.

Any delay in treatment of time-sensitive conditions may negatively impact on the patient, especially with neurologic emergencies such as ischemic stroke. Indeed, for every 30-minute delay in revascularization, a patient's risk of poor outcome increases by 10 percent.[8] Prehospital delay in transporting patients to a healthcare facility with signs of acute stroke may be a significant factor in the overall time delay in receiving definitive care.[9] When patients present with signs of posterior cerebral circulation insufficiency (dizziness, ataxia), this delay was even more pronounced. The stroke chapter in this book has additional information on the diagnosis and treatment of acute stroke.

Key challenges

Moderate-quality recommendations

To date, there are no rigorous studies indicating the ideal approach to evaluating and managing a patient with a chief complaint of dizziness in the prehospital setting. The multi-factorial nature of dizziness makes this condition difficult to study effectively. The challenge in approaching the dizzy patient is twofold. The first challenge is defining what the patient is experiencing and then determining whether the dizziness requires emergent evaluation and intervention. The ability to accurately determine whether dizziness is stemming from a life-threatening condition versus a benign one may not be possible given the limited time and resources available in the prehospital setting. Therefore, the EMS professional should have a low threshold to transport the patient to a facility where a more detailed work-up can be performed. Dizzy patients who are elderly, with multiple co-morbidities such as cardiovascular risk factors, diabetes, prior stroke or who present with focal neurologic findings on physical exam should be considered high-risk patients.

The EMS professional should focus on identifying life-threatening entities. These include:

- serious cardiac dysrhythmias or cardiac syncope;
- centrally mediated causes of vertigo;
- life-threatening metabolic/electrolyte derangements.

To identify these life-threats when evaluating a dizzy patient, the prehospital professional may enhance the standard history and physical by performing each of the following:

- blood glucose test;
- 12 lead ECG;
- focused neurologic exam (facial droop, slurred speech or pronator drift);
- focused cardiovascular exam measuring blood pressure from both arms and assessing peripheral pulses.

Most healthcare providers assign cardiovascular pathology to presyncope or syncope rather than vertigo. This tendency to rigidly group "dizziness" into vestibular and neurological causes and presyncope/syncope into cardiac causes may contribute to the lack of robust evidence linking cardiovascular etiology to dizziness. This practice discounts many significant cardiovascular causes for dizziness.

A systematic review evaluated how frequently cardiovascular disease presents as syncope.[10] Studies published between 1972 and 2007 were examined, and those available studies showed that about 10 percent of patients with primary cardiovascular disease experience dizziness as a dominant or presenting symptom.[11] Type A aortic dissection and sick sinus syndrome are examples of cardiovascular conditions that may present as dizziness.[12, 13, 14] Thus, the prehospital provider should perform a focused exam including cardiopulmonary exam, peripheral pulse evaluation, determination of blood pressure discrepancies between right and left upper extremities, and a screening 12 lead ECG if capable.

Early stroke detection is of utmost importance.[15] A retrospective review of 907 patients presenting with dizziness to a tertiary care medical center over a roughly two-year period was conducted to determine the rate and predictors for serious neurologic disease.[16] Five percent of patients had a serious neurologic diagnosis: most of these were found to have strokes. Factors found to be independently associated with serious neurologic disease were age over 60, chief complaint of imbalance or any focal neurologic deficit on exam. Reassuringly, an isolated finding of dizziness without any other factors was associated with a benign etiology for the patient's symptoms.

Metabolic and endocrine disorders are well-known entities that can elicit dizziness.[17, 18] Patients with a pre-existing history of diabetes are the obvious at-risk population, and finger stick blood glucose testing is a quick way to determine if the symptoms are caused by hypoglycemia or hyperglycemia.

Low-quality recommendations

Very few studies look at dizziness from the perspective of the prehospital setting. One retrospective study examined factors based on a brief history and physical exam that could predict which patients were likely to have a neurological cause of vertigo.[1] Several parameters were identified that could be used by paramedics to recognize central vertigo, typically a cerebellar stroke. In this study, 23 patients were transported by EMS to a teaching hospital between April 2011 and March 2012 with a chief complaint of vertigo. Of the 23 patients studied, four had strokes (two had cerebellar infarction and two had cerebellar hemorrhage) and 19 had peripheral vertigo. A systolic blood pressure above 160 mmHg and lack of horizontal component of nystagmus was predictive of central cerebellar stroke with 100 percent sensitivity and 84 percent specificity. This study was limited by the use of patients collected at a single center and small sample size.

A prospective cross-sectional study evaluated the use of a three-step oculomotor exam to determine whether central causes of vertigo could be identified based on exam and risk factors in 101 patients at an academic medical center.[6] The three-step oculomotor exam was 100 percent sensitive and 96 percent specific for detecting stroke. A major limiting factor is that the exams were conducted by highly specialized neuro-ophthalmology physicians in an in-patient or office setting. Feasibility of such an exam undertaken by non-physician providers is yet to be determined.

Orthostatic blood pressure measurement

Orthostatic hypotension refers to a sudden decrease in blood pressure that occurs when a patient moves to a standing position from the seated or supine position. Traditionally, this has been defined as a decrease of systolic blood pressure of at least 20 mmHg or decrease in diastolic blood pressure of at least 10 mmHg within 3 minutes of assuming the standing position.[19] Dizziness is the most common symptom reported when this precipitous drop in blood pressure occurs and is most commonly found in elderly patients.[20, 21] Routine determination of orthostatic vital signs has been proposed to evaluate dizzy patients. Utility of routine orthostatic vital signs in the prehospital setting is unclear.

Summary

Evaluation of the dizzy patient in the prehospital setting is a challenging task. To date, no clear guidelines exist on how prehospital providers should approach these patients. It seems prudent for the prehospital professional to remain vigilant and have low threshold to consider life-threatening causes of dizziness, since it is so challenging to differentiate between benign and malignant causes of vertigo in the field. To this end, it seems reasonable that the prehospital professional can focus on what can be performed feasibly in the field. Obtaining a blood glucose level, acquiring a 12 lead ECG and performing a focused physical exam may help identify a subgroup of patients with immediately life-threatening conditions.

Key issues for future investigation

The dizzy patient is a challenging chief complaint to address in any setting. Barriers to accurate diagnosis in the prehospital environment consist of a combination of limited time and resources to correctly determine whether their symptoms are due to a life-threatening or debilitating condition versus a more benign process at work.

The following specific questions need to be studied in the prehospital arena:

1. Is there a prehospital test or diagnostic tool that can accurately determine which patients who present with dizziness are due to central vestibular causes requiring emergent transport to a medical facility?
2. Which physical finding or available studies could best determine which patients in the prehospital setting are experiencing dizziness due to a life-threatening vascular insult?
3. In a tiered EMS system, is there a subset of patients who present with dizziness who should be transported by advanced life support units rather than basic life support units?

REFERENCES

1. Okada, M., Nakagawa, Y. and Inokuchi, S. (2012). "Out-of-hospital scaling to recognize central vertigo," *Tokai J. Exp. Clin. Med.* 37(3): 71–4.

2. Kentala, E. and Rauch, S. D. (2003). "A practical assessment algorithm for diagnosis of dizziness," *Otolaryngol. Head Neck Surg.* 128(1): 54–9.

3. Lee, T. H. (2012). "Diagnosing the cause of vertigo: A practical approach," *Hong Kong Med. J.* 18(4): 327–32.

4. "Vestibular system" (2013). Available at www.britannica. com/EBchecked/topic/175622/human-ear/65037/ Vestibular-system#ref531802.

5. Blotzer, J. W. and Henderson, M. C. (2012). "Syncope" in M. C. Henderson, L. M. Tierney and G. W. Smetana (eds.), *The Patient History: An Evidence-Based Approach to Differential Diagnosis*, 2nd edn (New York: McGraw-Hill), chapter 29.

6. Kattah, J. C., Talkad, A. V., Wang, D. Z. *et al.* (2009). "HINTS to diagnose stroke in the acute vestibular syndrome: Three-step bedside oculomotor examination more sensitive than early MRI diffusion-weighted imaging," *Stroke* 40(11): 3504–10.

7. Schneider, J. I. and Olshaker, J. S. (2012). "Vertigo, vertebrobasilar disease, and posterior circulation ischemic stroke," *Emerg. Med. Clin. North Am.* 30(3): 681–93.

8. Khatri, P., Abruzzo, T., Yeatts, S. D. *et al.* (2009). "Good clinical outcome after ischemic stroke with successful revascularization is time-dependent," *Neurology* 73(13): 1066–72.

9. Evenson, K., Foraker, R., Morris, D. *et al.* (2009). "A comprehensive review of prehospital and in-hospital delay times in acute stroke care," *International Journal of Stroke* 4(3): 187–99.

10. Newman-Toker, D. E., Dy, F. J., Stanton, V. *et al.* (2008). "How often is dizziness from primary cardiovascular disease true vertigo? A systematic review," *J. Gen. Intern. Med.* 23(12): 2087–94.

11. Culic, V., Miric, D. and Eterovic, D. (2001). "Correlation between symptomatology and site of acute myocardial infarction," *Int. J. Cardiol.* 77(2–3): 163–8.

12. Demiryoguran, N. S., Karcioglu, O., Topacoglu, H. *et al.* (2006). "Painless aortic dissection with bilateral carotid involvement presenting with vertigo as the chief complaint," *Emerg. Med. J.* 23(2): e15.

13. Newman-Toker, D. E. and Camargo, C. A. Jr. (2006). "'Cardiogenic vertigo' – true vertigo as the presenting manifestation of primary cardiac disease," *Nat. Clin. Pract. Neurol.* 2(3): 167–72.

14. Lee, E. W., Jourabachi, N., Sauk, S. C. *et al.* (2013). "Case report: an extensive Stanford type A aortic dissection involving bilateral carotid and iliac arteries," *Case Reports in Radiology*, Article ID: 607012.

15. Kothari, R. U., Pancioli, A., Liu, Y. *et al.* (1999). "Cincinnati Perhospital Stroke Scale: reproducibility and validity," *Ann. Emerg. Med.* 33(4): 373–8.

16. Navi, B. B., Kamel, H. and Kim, A. S. (2012). "Rate and predictors of serious neurologic causes of dizziness in the emergency department," *Mayo Clin. Proc.* 87(11): 1080–8.

17. Serra, A. P., de Carvalho Lopes, K., Dorigueto, R. S. *et al.* (2009). "Blood glucose and insulin levels in patients with peripheral vestibular disease," *Braz. J. Otorhinolaryngol.* 75(5): 701–5.

18. Fonseca, A. S., Angeleri, S. and Davidsohn, V. (2006). "Correlation between dizziness and impaired glucose metabolism," *Rev. Bras. Otorrinolaringol.* 72(3): 367–9.

19. Lanier, J. B., Mote, M. B. and Clay, E. C. (2011). "Evaluation and management of orthostatic hypotension," *Am. Fam. Physician* 84(5): 527–36.

20. Rutan, G. H., Hermanson, B. Bild, D. E. *et al.* (1992). "Orthostatic hypotension in older adults. The Cardiovascular Health Study. CHS Collaborative Research Group," *Hypertension* 19(6 Pt 1): 508–19.

21. Ooi, W. L., Barrett, S., Hossain, M. *et al.* (1997). "Patterns of orthostatic blood pressure change and their clinical correlates in a frail, elderly population," *JAMA* 277(16): 1299–304.

Chapter 2

Headache

Michael G. Millin and Jeffrey Kelly

Recommendations

High quality

There are insufficient data to support high-quality recommendations for this topic.

Moderate quality

1. Patients that present with a complaint of headache and fever, altered sensorium, vision changes or a headache described as new or the worst of life should be transported to an acute care facility for diagnostic evaluation to determine if there is a secondary, or pathologic, cause to the headache.
2. EMS providers should have knowledge of these pathologic causes of headaches so that they are able to adequately inform their patients to the risks of not getting emergent treatment when it is indicated.

Prehospital Care of Neurologic Emergencies, ed. Todd J. Crocco and Michael R. Sayre. Published by Cambridge University Press. © Cambridge University Press 2014.

3. EMS providers may consider the use of oxygen and anti-emetics for the treatment of headache as these treatment modalities have limited risk and have been found to be effective.

Low quality

1. EMS providers may consider the use of opioids and non-steroidal anti-inflammatory medications for the treatment of headaches. Although their use has been found to be effective for the management of headache, there are risks associated with their use. In addition, there is a paucity of literature related to the use of these medications for the management of headache in the EMS environment.

Overview

Although headaches are a common complaint for presentation to emergency care services, pathological diagnosis (or secondary causes) rates are quite low, averaging around 2 percent of all patients presenting with a headache.[1] Since the definitive diagnosis of the pathological causes of headaches is typically made by advanced testing, such as computed tomography, magnetic resonance imaging or lumbar puncture, it is likely that EMS providers will not be able to differentiate pathological from benign headaches. Therefore, EMS providers should assume that a patient with a headache has emergent pathology until proven otherwise.

Although EMS providers are unlikely to determine that a patient has a pathological process causing the patient's headache, an astute EMS provider, paying attention to key historical and physical findings, may be able to differentiate those patients that are at higher risk for pathological causes of the headache. This heightened awareness will be helpful for determining transport decisions, protecting EMS providers and the public from possible communicable diseases, and providing patients and families with accurate information in convincing patients to not refuse EMS care and transport.

Table 2.1 Headache signs and symptoms concerning for emergent pathology

History	Recent head trauma
	New or worsening headaches
	Sudden onset with maximal intensity in a minute of onset
	Triggered by Valsalva, exertion or sexual activity
	Pregnancy
	Age > 50
	Vision changes
	Fever
	Weight loss
	Immunocompromised state or history of cancer
Physical	Fever
	Seizures
	Focal neurological findings
	Weakness
	Altered mental status
	Inability to ambulate
	Stiff neck
	Unequal pupils

Evaluation of the headache patient begins with the historical exam. Historical findings of concern include: recent head trauma; new onset of headache or worsening of a pattern of existing headaches; sudden onset of headache with maximal intensity within a minute of onset of headache; headaches triggered by Valsalva, exertion or sexual activity; headaches during pregnancy; patient's age greater than 50; focal neurological signs including seizures, altered mental status, weakness or vision changes; and systemic illness including fevers or weight loss. EMS providers should also pay attention to headaches in patients with cancer or an immunocompromised state such as HIV or current treatment with immunosuppressant medications.[2]

Physical findings of concern associated with a headache include: unequal weakness; generalized malaise and inability to ambulate; fevers; neck stiffness; and unequal pupils.

Regardless of the cause of the headache and the level of concern of the EMS providers that the cause is related to emergent pathology, EMS provider management of headaches is essentially the same. Patients with concern for infectious causes of headache should be transported using isolation precautions with respiratory isolation masks and post-exposure prophylaxis when appropriate. The use of anti-emetics has been shown to be effective in the management of headaches, and certainly is a benign treatment that may help to facilitate a safe transport. Other treatment modalities may be considered on a case-by-case basis.

Key challenges

Causes of headaches – primary (benign)

Tension

The tension-type headache is the most common type of headache, with prevalence as high as 78 percent. This type of headache is suspected to originate via both peripheral and central pain mechanisms.[3] Patients experiencing a tension-type headache will present with vague symptoms: the pain will be generalized, but most intense near the occiput and the posterior neck. Tension headaches are most commonly provoked by stress or fatigue. External auditory or visual stimuli may also trigger a tension headache. A tension-type headache will not cause focal neurological symptoms.[4] Due to the vague nature of this headache, the diagnosis of tension headache is often made after ruling out secondary causes to the headache.

Migraine

Although migraine is a common cause of headache presentation to emergency services, like tension headaches, its actual diagnosis depends on meeting certain criteria as established by the International Classification of Headache Disorders (ICHD), which conclude with the statement that the headache is not attributed to another disorder.[4, 5] Migraine headaches typically last 4 to 72 hours, are unilateral, often associated with nausea and/or vomiting, and may or may not be associated with an aura consisting of fully reversible visual, sensory or speech disturbances. Patients often present to emergency care with first or worst headache or a headache that is their "last straw," typically necessitating extensive work-ups to look for secondary causes of headache.[6]

Cluster

The cause of cluster headache is uncertain. Although traumatic brain injury and anatomical changes are thought to be involved, more research is required to determine whether the relationship is more than a random association.[7, 8] Cluster headaches tend to be more prevalent in men and are characterized by severe unilateral, orbital, supraorbital or temporal pain lasting from 15 minutes to 3 hours. To meet criteria set forth in the ICHD, patients must have five episodes with a frequency rate of one every other day to eight per day.[4] Patients also experience one of the following symptoms during the episode: ipsilateral redness or tearing of the eyes, nasal congestion or rhinorrhea, eyelid edema, perspiration on the forehead or face, pinpoint pupil or ptosis, or agitation or restlessness.

Caffeine withdrawal

Caffeine is a frequently used psychostimulant, which has effective properties for the treatment of primary headaches for individuals who consume low and/or infrequent quantities. For those who consume caffeine on a regular basis, caffeine withdrawal may often precipitate the onset of a headache. The symptoms of caffeine withdrawal headache may often be confused for a migraine headache as they appear with severe headache, fatigue, nausea and vomiting. Symptoms often resolve with consumption of caffeine.[9]

Causes of headaches – secondary (pathologic)

Infectious

A new-onset headache occurring at the same time as other symptoms concerning for possible infection should be assumed to be secondary headache caused by meningitis until proven otherwise. Since the definitive diagnosis for meningitis is made from fluid collected by lumbar puncture, EMS providers will only discover that a patient has meningitis through hospital follow-up care. Of note, the Ryan Act protects EMS providers by ensuring that there are no road blocks to dissemination of information to EMS providers regarding possible exposure to bacterial meningitis.[4, 10]

Meningitis should be suspected when a patient presents with headache, neck stiffness and fever. The patient may also complain of nausea, vomiting and photophobia.[11] Although commonly thought to be helpful in the clinical diagnosis of meningitis, Thomas *et al.* found Kernig's sign and Brudzinski's sign to have little diagnostic value in assessing for meningitis.[12] Even after adequate treatment with antibiotics, a headache with the preceding characteristics lasting for more than three months is known as a chronic post-bacterial meningitis headache.[4]

Other types of infections can cause headache. The ICHD defines headaches caused by abscess, empyema, HIV/AIDS and systemic infections.[4] Because of the difficulty with pinpointing the cause of a headache, providers should encourage patients to be transported to the hospital and undergo a thorough assessment.

EMS providers often question the need for emergent post-exposure prophylaxis when in contact with a patient with suspected meningitis. Interestingly, *Neisseria meningitidis*, the bacterial agent of most concern in terms of the need for post-exposure prophylaxis, rarely results in transmission to emergency care providers when proper precautions are taken.[10] EMS providers in contact with a patient with a headache and fever should transport the patient using universal precautions with a focus on droplet precautions. The risk to EMS providers is the greatest when exposed to respiratory droplets while involved in airway management.

Post-exposure prophylaxis for meningitis typically includes two days of treatment with rifampin (600 mg twice a day) or ciprofloxacin and ceftriaxone for those unable to complete a course of rifampin.[10] EMS providers should contact their infection control officer and/or medical director for specific advice after a possible exposure.

Subarachnoid hemorrhage (SAH)

According to a review by Edlow *et al.*, SAH accounts for about 1 percent of patients presenting to emergency departments complaining of headache.[13] Providers should be concerned for spontaneous SAH in a patient with a history of abrupt onset headache associated with vomiting, syncope or a complaint of a stiff neck. Since approximately 50 percent of patients with SAH present with only a mild headache or a headache of sudden onset that is in resolution, emergency care providers need to have a heightened sense of awareness for the potential of missing SAH, which can result in severe consequences for the patient.[13]

Ophthalmologic

Headaches associated with eye complaints may or may not be related to pathology directly related to the eye. Patients may complain of excessive eye tearing (lacrimation), blurry vision, swelling of the eye or direct pain in the eye. Providers should consider emergencies related to the eye, including acute glaucoma and iritis, and any intracranial emergency that may produce increased intracranial pressure (ICP), including idiopathic intracranial hypertension, aneurysmal and dissection emergencies, and space-occupying lesions.[14] All headaches associated with a complaint of vision changes warrant emergent evaluation.

Neoplastic

Headache in a patient with a known history of intracranial tumor should always be considered of potential concern for any pathology that may result in increased ICP such as increasing tumor size or new metastatic lesions, intracranial bleeding or obstructive hydrocephalus.[15] Much more challenging for the emergency care provider is headache in a patient with an undiagnosed tumor. Headaches described with a new diagnosis of intracranial tumors are typically a result of increased ICP and classically described as severe, constant, progressive pain worsening upon waking and associated with nausea and vomiting.[15]

Treatment

Patients often initially self-treat their headaches with over-the-counter medications using combinations of aspirin, acetaminophen and caffeine.[16] Healthcare providers may find the same "cocktail" of medications to be useful in the treatment of patients with headaches.[17] Supplementing ibuprofen for aspirin has also been found to be helpful.[16, 18] If the initial barrage of medications are ineffective, the provider may follow up with anti-emetics. High concentrations of inhaled oxygen have also been found to have utility for the treatment of headaches with minimal side effects. In general, secondary headaches tend to improve as the underlying cause of the headache is treated. The following provides a review of the common treatment options for the management of headache in the EMS environment.

Oxygen

Although high concentrations of inhaled oxygen have been found to be effective for treating both migraine and cluster headaches, a case review found a recurrence of migraine symptoms after the patient resumed breathing normoxic air.[19, 20] A review by Francis *et al.* found high-level evidence for reduction of pain related to cluster headache when oxygen was administered with triptans.[21] Some evidence suggests that high-flow oxygen may be effective in reducing pain for all headache types,[22] although caution should be exercised to not

Table 2.2 Headache treatment

Class	Medication	Route / dosage	Benefits	Disadvantages
Opiod	morphine	0.1 mg/kg IV, IM	Effective Ease of administration	Rebound Dependence Mental status depression
	fentanyl	1 mcg/kg IV, IM, IN		
Anti-emetic	metoclopramide prochlorperazine	10–20 mg IV 20 mg IV	No additional risk of hemorrhage Few side effects	Must be combined with other agents
Oxygen	oxygen	6–15 lpm NRM	Ease of administration Broad sprectrum of effectiveness Low cost Few side effects	Caution in treatment of headache with suspected stroke

NSAIDS	ketorolac ibuprofen naproxen	30 mg IV/IM 600 mg po 825 mg po	Non-sedative Ease of administration Few side effects	May be associated with intracranial bleeding Not as effective as other treatments
Other OTC pain med.	aspirin acetaminophen	500–1,000 mg po 500–1,000 mg po	Ease of administration Low cost	Unknown risk of intracranial bleeding
Combination	aspirin/ acetaminophen/ caffeine	500/400/50 mg po	Ease of administration Low cost	Disadvantages of the individual components
Triptan	sumatriptan zolmitriptan	6 mg sc 5–10 mg nasal spray	Effective	More costly and more side effects when compared to equally effective options

create a hyperoxic state in patients with headache of unknown origin when stroke is suspected.[23]

Anti-emetics

Anti-emetics work alone or in combination with other agents to reduce symptoms associated with headache. Ondansetron may be effective in reducing nausea, but because a mild to moderate headache is associated as a side effect of ondansetron, other anti-emetics should be considered.[24]

Metoclopramide (20 mg) with diphenhydramine (25 mg) has been found to be more effective than ketorolac for managing tension and recurring headache.[25] When combined with aspirin or acetaminophen, 10 mg of metoclopramide is as effective as sumatriptan, perhaps with fewer side effects.[26]

Both promethazine (25 mg) and prochlorperazine (20 mg) have successfully been used as single agents for headache management. While both are equally effective for managing the symptoms, prochlorperazine works faster and causes less drowsiness.[27]

Opioid

Opioids have long been considered to be effective and their use is widespread for the treatment of headache.[28–30] Although opioids are often found to be no more effective than the anti-emetics, with refractory headaches they may provide the patient with significant relief and they have been found to be superior to placebo. The risk with using opioid medications to treat headache is that they have been associated with being a cause for rebound headaches, they have the potential to result in drug dependency, they are often a cause of medication overuse headache, and their mental status depressive side effect may make it difficult for further assessment of the patient by other healthcare providers.[31-4]

NSAIDS and other simple analgesics

In general, nonsteroidal anti-inflammatory drugs (NSAIDS) may be more effective than simple analgesics. Ibuprofen at 800 mg and naproxen sodium at 825 mg are the top choices for treatment of tension-type headache; both have few side effects.[16] Ketorolac reduces symptoms, but not as effectively as other treatments for recurrent and tension headaches.[25] NSAIDs temporarily and reversibly inhibit platelet function and may foster bleeding.[35] Despite this, patients using these drugs generally tend to have a low risk of morbidity due to hemorrhagic stroke.[36] The literature on the safety of ketorolac and intracranial hemorrhage, however, is mixed and warrants further investigation.[37]

Other

If migraine or cluster headache is not successfully treated after the initial barrage of simple analgesics and NSAIDs, the provider may follow up with triptans and/or dihydroergotamine, although these medications are seldom carried by EMS providers.[19] These drugs function by causing intracranial vasoconstriction. There is high-level evidence that a combination of 6 mg of subcutaneous sumatriptan, 5 to 10 mg of nasal zolmitriptan and high-flow oxygen are effective in reducing pain.[21] Sumatriptan is also available as a nasal spray; it is more effective than nasal dihydroergotamine and has fewer side effects.[38]

Sumatriptan more frequently has side effects, minor as they may be, when compared to simple analgesics.[26]

Be aware that medication overuse can lead to rebound headaches. In this case, migraine prevention is preferred.[39]

Until recently, there was insufficient evidence to draw a conclusion on the role of acupuncture in headache management. Acupuncture may be beneficial for both tension and migraine headache,[40, 41] although its use in the EMS environment is less than practical.

Summary

Although the greater majority of patients who present to emergency care for a headache do not have a pathological reason for their headache that is of acute emergent concern, it is often difficult to determine solely by history and physical exam that emergent pathology does not exist. Further, since the definitive diagnosis for these pathological causes of headache often require advanced diagnostics that are not available in the EMS environment (i.e. computed tomography, magnetic resonance imaging and analysis of cerebral spinal fluid via a lumbar puncture), EMS providers must have a heightened level of concern for the causes of headaches that require emergent treatment.

Any patient presenting to emergency care providers with headache should prompt transport to an acute care facility for further diagnostic evaluation. Patients that should give the EMS provider the greatest concern are those patients with fever, altered sensorium, vision changes, and a complaint of new or worst headache.

Key issues for future investigation

In general, the area of headache evaluation and management in the EMS environment needs further study. Recommendations made in this chapter are all based on studies from other settings, as there is a paucity of literature on the EMS management of headaches. Perhaps most importantly, further study on headache patients who refuse EMS treatment and transport resulting in them having emergent pathology would help EMS providers in understanding the importance of recognizing the emergent risks with this complaint. Further study on the benefits and side effects of treatment modalities for headache in the EMS environment would also be of value.

REFERENCES

1. Goldstein, J. N., Camargo, C. A. Jr., Pelletier, A. J. *et al.* (2006). "Headache in United States emergency departments: demographics, work-up and frequency of pathological diagnoses," *Cephalalgia* 26(6): 684–90.

2. De Luca, G. C. and Bartleson, J. D. (2010). "When and how to investigate the patient with headache," *Semin. Neurol.* 30(2): 131–44.

3. Aminoff, M. (2005). "Nervous System" in ed. L. Tierney, S. McPhee and M. Papadakis (eds.), *Current Medical Diagnosis and Treatment*, 44th edn. (New York: Lange Medical Books/McGraw-Hill).

4. Headache Classification Subcommittee of the International Headache Society (2004). "The International Classification of Headache Disorders 2nd edition," *Cephalalgia* 24(Suppl. 1): 9–160.

5. Mathew, P. G. and Garza, I. (2011). "Headache," *Semin. Neurol.* 31(1): 5–17.

6. Friedman, B. W. and Grosberg, B. M. (2009). "Diagnosis and management of the primary headache disorders in the emergency department setting," *Emerg. Med. Clin. North Am.* 27(1): 71–87, viii.

7. Lambru, G. and Matharu, M. (2012). "Traumatic head injury in cluster headache: cause or effect?" *Curr. Pain Headache Rep.* 16(2): 162–9.

8. Seifert, C. L., Magon, S., Staehle, K. *et al.* (2012). "A case-control study on cortical thickness in episodic cluster headache," *Headache* 52(9): 1362–8.

9. Shapiro, R. E. (2007). "Caffeine and headaches," *Neurol. Sci.* 28(Suppl. 2): S179–83.

10. Bolyard, E. A., Tablan, O. C., Williams, W. W. *et al.* (1998). "Guideline for infection control in healthcare personnel, 1998. Hospital Infection Control Practices Advisory Committee," *Infect. Control Hosp. Epidemiol.* 19(6): 407–63.

11. Davis, L. E. and Katzman, J. G. (2008). "Chronic daily headache: when to suspect meningitis," *Curr. Pain Headache Rep.* 12(1): 50–5.

12. Thomas, K. E., Hasbun, R., Jekel, J. *et al.* (2002). "The diagnostic accuracy of Kernig's sign, Brudzinski's sign, and nuchal rigidity in adults with suspected meningitis," *Clin. Infect. Dis.* 35(1): 46–52.

13. Edlow, J. A., Malek, A. M. and Ogilvy, C. S. (2008). "Aneurysmal subarachnoid hemorrhage: update for emergency physicians," *J. Emerg. Med.* 34(3): 237–51.

14. Friedman, D. I. (2008). "Headache and the eye," *Curr. Pain Headache Rep.* 12(4): 296–304.

15. Goldlust, S. A., Graber, J. J., Bossert, D. F. *et al.* (2010). "Headache in patients with cancer," *Curr. Pain Headache Rep.* 14(6): 455–64.

16. Fumal, A. and Schoenen, J. (2008). "Tension-type headache: current research and clinical management," *Lancet Neurol.* 7(1): 70–83.

17. Diener, H. C., Peil, H. and Aicher, B. (2011). "The efficacy and tolerability of a fixed combination of acetylsalicylic acid, paracetamol, and caffeine in patients with severe headache: a post-hoc subgroup analysis from a multicentre, randomized, double-blind, single-dose, placebo-controlled parallel group study," *Cephalalgia* 31(14): 1466–76.

18. Rabbie, R., Derry, S. and Moore, R. A. (2013). "Ibuprofen with or without an antiemetic for acute migraine headaches in adults," *Cochrane Database Syst. Rev.* 4: CD008039.

19. Jurgens, T. P., Schulte, L. H. and May, A. (2013). "Oxygen treatment is effective in migraine with autonomic symptoms," *Cephalalgia* 33(1): 65–7.

20. Cohen, A. S., Burns, B. and Goadsby, P. J. (2009). "High-flow oxygen for treatment of cluster headache: a randomized trial," *JAMA* 302(22): 2451–7.

21. Francis, G. J., Becker, W. J. and Pringsheim, T. M. (2010). "Acute and preventive pharmacologic treatment of cluster headache," *Neurology* 75(5): 463–73.

22. Ozkurt, B., Cinar, O., Cevik, E. *et al.* (2012). "Efficacy of high-flow oxygen therapy in all types of headache: a prospective, randomized, placebo-controlled trial," *Am. J. Emerg. Med.* 30(9): 1760–4.

23. Millin, M. G., Gullett, T. and Daya, M. R. (2007). "EMS management of acute stroke – out-of-hospital treatment and stroke system development (resource document to NAEMSP position statement)," *Prehosp. Emerg. Care* 11(3): 318–25.

24. Patka, J., Wu, D. T., Abraham, P. *et al.* (2011). "Randomized controlled trial of ondansetron vs. prochlorperazine in adults in the emergency department," *West J. Emerg. Med.* 12(1): 1–5.

25. Friedman, B. W., Adewunmi, V., Campbell, C. *et al.* (2013). "A randomized trial of intravenous ketorolac versus intravenous metoclopramide plus diphenhydramine for tension-type and all nonmigraine, noncluster recurrent headaches," *Ann. Emerg. Med.* (e-pub. ahead of print).

26. Kirthi, V., Derry, S., Moore, R. A. *et al.* (2010). "Aspirin with or without an antiemetic for acute migraine headaches in adults," *Cochrane Database Syst. Rev.* 4: CD008041.

27. Callan, J. E., Kostic, M. A., Bachrach, E. A. *et al.* (2008). "Prochlorperazine vs. promethazine for headache treatment in the emergency department: a randomized controlled trial," *J. Emerg. Med.* 35(3): 247–53.

28. Kelley, N. E. and Tepper, D. E. (2012). "Rescue therapy for acute migraine, part 1: triptans, dihydroergotamine, and magnesium," *Headache* 52(1): 114–28.

29. Landy, S. H. (2004). "Oral transmucosal fentanyl citrate for the treatment of migraine headache pain in outpatients: a case series," *Headache* 44(8): 762–6.

30. Friedman, B. W., Kapoor, A., Friedman, M. S. *et al.* (2008). "The relative efficacy of meperidine for the treatment of acute migraine: a meta-analysis of randomized controlled trials," *Ann. Emerg. Med.* 52(6): 705–13.

31. Tepper, S. J. and Tepper, D. E. (2010). "Breaking the cycle of medication overuse headache," *Cleve. Clin. J. Med.* 77(4): 236–42.

32. Bigal, M. E. and Lipton, R. B. (2008). "Excessive acute migraine medication use and migraine progression," *Neurology* 71(22): 1821–8.

33. Ward, T. N. (2008). "Drug-induced refractory headache," *Headache* 48(5): 728, discussion 729.

34. Von Korff, M. Galer, B. S. and Stang, P. (1995). "Chronic use of symptomatic headache medications," *Pain* 62(2): 179–86.

35. Schafer, A. I. (1999). "Effects of nonsteroidal anti-inflammatory therapy on platelets," *Am. J. Med.* 106(5B): 25S–36S.

36. Choi, N. K., Park, B. J., Jeong, S. W. *et al.* (2008). "Nonaspirin nonsteroidal anti-inflammatory drugs and hemorrhagic stroke risk: the Acute Brain Bleeding Analysis study," *Stroke* 39(3): 845–9.

37. Magni, G., La Rosa, I., Melillo, G. *et al.* (2013). "Intracranial hemorrhage requiring surgery in neurosurgical patients given ketorolac: a case-control study within a cohort (2001–2010)," *Anesth. Analg.* 116(2): 443–7.

38. Boureau, F., Kappos, L., Schoenen, J. *et al.* (2000). "A clinical comparison of sumatriptan nasal spray and dihydroergotamine nasal spray in the acute treatment of migraine," *Int. J. Clin. Pract.* 54(5): 281–6.

39. Silberstein, S. D. (2000). "Practice parameter: evidence-based guidelines for migraine headache (an evidence-based review): report of the Quality Standards Subcommittee of the American Academy of Neurology," *Neurology* 55(6): 754–62.

40. Schiapparelli, P., Allais, G., Rolando, S. *et al.* (2011). "Acupuncture in primary headache treatment," *Neurol. Sci.* 32(Suppl. 1): S15–18.

41. Linde, K., Allais, G., Brinkhaus, B. *et al.* (2009). "Acupuncture for migraine prophylaxis," *Cochrane Database Syst. Rev.* 1: CD001218.

Chapter 3

Seizures

Robert Silbergleit and M. Kay Vonderschmidt

Recommendations

High quality

1. Patients with generalized convulsive seizures that continue (or that rapidly recur without awakening) for longer than 5 minutes should rapidly receive adequate doses of benzodiazepines. Such patients should be considered to be in status epilepticus.[1, 2]

2. For patients who do not have intravenous (IV) access established, intramuscular (IM) midazolam can be administered more rapidly and is at least as effective as intravenous lorazepam at stopping seizures.[3]

3. In children, lorazepam is as effective as diazepam for the initial treatment of status epilepticus.

Prehospital Care of Neurologic Emergencies, ed. Todd J. Crocco and Michael R. Sayre. Published by Cambridge University Press. © Cambridge University Press 2014.

Moderate quality

1. Isolated, self-limited, breakthrough seizures in patients with known seizure disorders generally do not require treatment with a benzodiazepine or other interventions.[4]

2. Give appropriate doses of benzodiazepines to patients who have ongoing seizures.[3, 5–9]

    (a) In adults, initiate treatment with midazolam 10 mg IM, or lorazepam 4 mg IV, or diazepam 10 mg IV.

    (b) In children (2 to 12 years or 13 to 40 kg), initiate treatment with midazolam 5 mg IM, or lorazepam 2 mg IV, or diazepam 5 mg IV (or at any age, lorazepam 0.1 mg/kg IV or diazepam 0.2 mg/kg IV). Children over 12 years of age or 40 kg body weight can also receive the same doses as adults.

    (c) For adults and children, repeat the initial dose if convulsions persist 10 minutes after drug administration.

3. Intranasal and buccal routes of administration of midazolam are similar in effectiveness to IM administration, and are preferable to rectal diazepam when intravenous access is not readily available.[10–13]

Low quality

1. Because the best supportive care during status epilepticus is to stop the seizure, definitive therapy with benzodiazepines should generally precede other interventions.[9]

2. Because the physiologic manifestions of the post-ictal period are generally transient and benign, most patients without other underlying problems can be managed with observation immediately after cessation of seizures.[9]

3. Patients with prolonged seizure symptoms without awakening that are suspected to be "pseudo-seizure" should usually be treated with benzodiazepines in the same manner as any other seizure patient, since the diagnosis of non-epileptic events can be challenging in the emergency setting.[9, 14]

Overview

Seizures are a common cause of EMS activation. In an analysis of San Francisco EMS dispatch, seizure was the seventh most common complaint, accounting for 6 percent of the total call volume, averaging more than 10 calls per day, and consistent with other reports.[15] Seizures are the result of sudden, usually brief, excessive synchronized electrical discharges in a group of brain cells (neurons). These discharges can occur in different parts of the brain or across the entire brain. Different patients may have different seizure symptoms depending on the location in the brain these discharges occur.

Seizures are not really a disease per se, but rather a manifestation of some underlying pathology. Patients with any number of underlying disorders or injuries characterized by recurrent seizures are considered to have epilepsy. Such patients generally require long-term treatment with anti-epileptic drugs.[16] Isolated, uncomplicated and self-limited seizures in patients with a known seizure disorder are the most frequent presentation of seizure. Such patients require little prehospital care and may not require transportation. A change in pattern or increasing frequency of seizures in patients with known seizure disorder, however, may be indicative of a dangerous acute pathology requiring emergency medical care. Patients with new onset seizures also require an emergent evaluation to determine, if possible, the underlying cause of the seizure – even if the seizure is brief and stops by itself.

Status epilepticus (SE) is defined as persistent or rapidly recurring seizures lasting for more than 5 minutes that generally do not stop by themselves. SE is a life-threatening medical emergency. While SE is much less common than self-limited seizures, there are at least 120,000 to 200,000 cases per year in the United States; and there are 55,000 annual deaths in patients with SE.[17-21] Prolonged seizures are associated with cardiorespiratory dysfunction (including aspiration, apnea and hypotension), metabolic derangements (including hyperthermia and acidosis) and direct excitotoxic neuronal cell death (causing irreversible brain injury). The most common causes of SE include non-compliance with anti-epileptic drugs in patients with seizure disorders, withdrawal from alcohol or certain medications, hypoglycemia or certain electrolyte abnormalities, neurotrauma, toxic exposures and infections, ischemia or other lesions within the central nervous system.[15]

EMS management

Most generalized convulsive seizures are isolated self-limited events, but when they do not stop spontaneously, they are a life-threatening neurological emergency needing immediate treatment.

Rapid administration of adequate doses of benzodiazepines is effective at stopping convulsions prior to emergency department arrival and decreasing the likelihood of both hospital and intensive care unit admission.[1, 3] The best available data suggest that intramuscular midazolam is the most effective route and agent in the prehospital setting (see "Key challenges," below).[3] Prehospital treatment also involves supportive care (prevention of further injury, airway and ventilatory assistance, supplemental oxygen, administration of glucose, etc.) during both the convulsions and the post-ictal state. EMS professionals should evaluate the patient for potentially life-threatening, treatable causes of seizure (such as hypoglycemia, arrhythmia or brain injury). Psychogenic non-epileptic spells (pseudo-seizures) are challenging to diagnose in any setting and should be an EMS diagnosis in only the most extreme and obvious presentation.[14]

Any patient with an ongoing seizure or persistent altered mental status after a seizure needs to be assessed for a treatable cause, such as hypoglycemia, hypoxia or hypotension. Paramedics should also consider and look for symptoms and signs beyond the seizure that may indicate other syndromes in the differential diagnosis such as stroke, myocardial infarction, toxic exposures, trauma, sepsis and withdrawal, as these may affect the optimal receiving hospital in systems with regionalized specialty care.

In patients with a new-onset simple self-limited generalized convulsive seizure, management by EMS includes excluding other life-threatening conditions, preparing for a recurrence and transporting the patient to an ED to facilitate careful evaluation for the specific cause. Most often, a cause is not found in the ED; and in most such cases, the patient never has another seizure.[22, 23] Others will develop recurrent seizures and be diagnosed with epilepsy. The most frequent etiologies discovered during ED evaluation are an adverse medication or illicit drug reaction, or withdrawal from a medication, illicit drug or alcohol. In children under 5 years of age, the most common cause of simple self-limited seizure is fever. Isolated febrile seizures are almost always benign. Febrile SE is uncommon, but is a serious issue when it occurs.

In patients with a simple self-limited seizure who have epilepsy, the cause is typically referred to as a breakthrough seizure. Management by EMS is similar to that of patients with new onset seizure. Such breakthroughs are most often caused by subtherapeutic anticonvulsant therapy from missed doses or changes in prescribed therapy or are idiopathic. Occasionally, breakthrough seizures reflect lowering of the seizure threshold by some other acute pathology or infection or are caused by withdrawal from alcohol or other substances. Some of these patients may not require transport.

Characterizing seizures

A good description of seizure activity witnessed prior to ED arrival is important in confirming the diagnosis and guiding therapy. EMS providers should interview witnesses at the scene to obtain details about the character and duration of the seizure, any prodromal symptoms, any urinary incontinence, and the character and duration of the post-ictal phase. EMS providers should also be able to identify and describe seizures that they witness. EMS calls are most often for generalized convulsive seizures. Generalized (grand mal) seizures often begin with the perception of an aura by the patient, which may be a smell, taste, sound or other sensation. This is followed by the sudden onset of convulsions in an ictal stage. This most often includes tonic (flexion or extension of the head, trunk or extremities) and then the clonic (rhythmic motor jerking of the extremities) activity. Patients are unconscious during these generalized tonic–clonic convulsions. The post-ictal phase is characterized by diminished consciousness, slowing and confusion, which usually resolves or improves over 15 to 30 minutes, but which can sometimes be prolonged for hours. Persistent post-ictal unconciousness after generalized seizure is concerning for ongoing subtle or non-convulsive generalized seizure activity. Focal neurological symptoms in the post-ictal period such as unilateral weakness should be noted. These may be a transient consequence of the seizure itself (Todd's phenomena) or may represent an underlying stroke or other acute pathology precipitating the seizure. Generalized convulsive status epilepticus is responsible for almost all the immediately life-threatening presentations of seizures.

Other types of seizures include focal or partial seizures. Focal seizures are unilateral manifestations of synchronized abnormal discharges limited to a specific area in the brain.

Patients with focal tonic–clonic seizures are typically conscious with uncontrolled jerking or movements in one body part. Complex partial seizures, temporal lobe seizures, petit mal and absence seizures are non-convulsive syndromes that may manifest as confusion, abrupt interruptions in fluent cognition or other behavioral changes. Patients may exhibit highly suggestive automatisms (lip smacking, fumbling with the hands), but these seizures are challenging to diagnose without electroencephalography (EEG).[24] Although they warrant urgent evaluation, these seizure disorders are unlikely to be immediately life-threatening.

On scene approach

Prevent further trauma by moving items such as tables and chairs out of the way of the seizing patient. Look for a medical ID bracelet while performing a rapid patient assessment.

Maintain an open airway with a nasal airway, measure oxygen saturation with a pulse oximeter and place the patient on oxygen by nasal cannula or non-rebreather mask if the oxygen saturation is below 94 percent. Measure the patient's blood glucose level and treat all patients with finger stick glucose below 60 mg/dl with 50 percent dextrose (D50) or glucagon. Provide cervical spine stabilization if injury is suspected as the precipitant or the result of the seizure.

Provide definitive EMS care by rapidly administering adequately dosed benzodiazepines and supportive care when required. Place the patient on a cardiac monitor. Hypoxic or hypoventilatory seizure patients with pinpoint pupils and other features of severe opiod toxidrome may be treated with naloxone. Before leaving, look around the scene for clues such as medication bottles or chemical exposures to the patient that may give an indication as to the etiology. Transport to an appropriate receiving facility.

Key challenges

High-quality recommendations

1. Patients with generalized convulsive seizures that continue (or that rapidly recur without awakening) for longer than 5 minutes should rapidly receive adequate doses of benzodiazepines. Such patients should be considered to be in status epilepticus.[1, 2]
2. For patients who do not have intravenous (IV) access established, intramuscular (IM) midazolam can be administered more rapidly and is at least as effective as intravenous lorazepam at stopping seizures.[3]
3. In children, lorazepam is as effective as diazepam for the initial treatment of status epilepticus.

Studies

The Prehospital Treatment of Status Epilepticus (PHTSE) Trial was conducted by Dr. Lowenstein and colleagues at the University of California, San Francisco in the late 1990s.[1, 25] PHTSE was a National Institute of Neurological Disorders and Stroke (NINDS) funded, randomized, controlled trial of diazepam, lorazepam and placebo in the prehospital treatment of status epilepticus (SE). After confirmation with a base physician, San Francisco paramedics enrolled 258 adult patients with generalized SE that had been seizing for more than 5 minutes. Subjects received one of three treatments: an initial dose of intravenous lorazepam 2 mg, intravenous diazepam 5 mg or an identical appearing intravenous placebo. An identical repeat dose was delivered in patients still seizing after 4 minutes for a total prehospital dose of up to 4 mg of IV lorazepam, and up to 10 mg IV diazepam or matching placebo. Paramedics were blinded to the treatment given. Convulsions had terminated at arrival to the ED in 59 percent of those treated with lorazepam, 43 percent of those treated with diazepam and only 21 percent of those treated with placebo. Importantly, the trial showed that early termination of seizures was associated with better clinical outcomes. Patients still convulsing on ED arrival were more likely to require admission to hospital and to the intensive care unit than those whose seizures were terminated before arrival at the hospital (73 vs. 32 percent). While both diazepam and lorazepam were more effective than placebo in PHTSE, the trial also suggested that IV lorazepam may be more effective than IV diazepam. However, lorazepam was thought to require refrigerated storage; and there were few data on the use of lorazepam by rectal or other non-intravenous routes of administration. As a result, diazepam remained the primary EMS benzodiazepine for treatment of SE after the PHSTE trial.

The Rapid Anticonvulsant Medication Prior to Arrival Trial (RAMPART) was conducted by the Neurological Emergencies Treatment Trials network from 2009 to 2011 at EMS sites across the United States.[3] RAMPART was an NINDS-funded, randomized, controlled trial of IM midazolam versus IV lorazepam given by paramedics to 893 adult and pediatric patients with generalized status epilepticus lasting longer than 5 minutes. The trial was conducted because some EMS systems began to use non-intravenous routes of midazolam instead of either lorazepam or diazepam. Midazolam was a putative optimal agent based on its ease of use, its stability, and some scant evidence on its effectiveness in the ED treatment of SE and the prehospital treatment of other conditions. RAMPART was designed to determine if IM midazolam was as safe and effective as the best IV therapy, lorazepam. In a blinded, double-dummy design, paramedics, operating without base physician communication, rapidly administered 10 mg of IM midazolam to adults and larger children (or 5 mg to younger children) plus an IV placebo, or an IM placebo plus 4 mg of IV lorazepam to adults or larger children (or 2 mg to younger children). All patients therefore received active treatment of their seizure. Patients receiving IM midazolam had termination of seizures prior to arrival in the ED 73 percent of the time, as compared to 63 percent in those receiving IV lorazepam. Although the trial was only designed to see if IM midazolam was non-inferior to IV lorazepam, it actually demonstrated that the IM route was superior to the IV route. The study also confirmed that lorazepam degrades in routine EMS drug storage in a manner that is both time and temperature dependent and should be restocked after about 60 days of EMS storage in the field unless refrigerated.[26]

The Pediatric Seizure Study was conducted by the Pediatric Emergency Care Applied Research Network from 2008 to 2012 at sites across the United States.[27] It was a National Institute of Child Health and Human Development (NICHD) funded, randomized, controlled trial of IV lorazepam versus IV diazepam in children with status epilepticus treated in the emergency department when not treated with IV benzodiazepines by paramedics. Children with more than 5 minutes of generalized status epilepticus were randomized to 0.1 mg/kg of lorazepam (maximum dose 4 mg) or 0.2 mg/kg of diazepam (maximum dose 8 mg). Half of this dose was repeated in 5 minutes if the patient was still convulsing. The investigators hypothesized that lorazepam would be more effective, but the rates of termination of seizure at 10 minutes post treatment were similar between the two study arms.

Second-line anticonvulsant medications (such as fosphenytoin, phenobarbital, valproate or levitiracetam) are used in the emergency department for patients with status epilepticus who remain refractory to adequate doses of benzodiazepines, but these agents generally require a slow IV load given over 10 to 20 minutes, and there are no trials of these agents in prehospital care.[9]

Moderate-quality recommendations

1. *Isolated, self-limited, breakthrough seizures in patients with known seizure disorders generally do not require treatment with a benzodiazepine or other interventions.* Most seizures are benign, self-limited events in patients with a known

history of epilepsy. Most patients with epilepsy do not activate EMS for these events when they occur at home, but EMS activation is common when such events occur in public. As long as patients are waking normally from the post-ictal state and are not having a pattern of rapidly recurring seizures, immediate treatment with a benzodiazepine is not indicated. If a patient with known epilepsy is waking normally, has no injuries from the event and is not having an accelerating pattern of seizures, it is common and reasonable for the patient to decline transport.

2. *Avoid initial underdosing of benzodiazepines in patients who are still seizing.* Seizures become increasingly refractory to therapy over time. Failing to give enough benzodiazepine initially may result in the need for much higher total doses or may contribute to the seizures becoming entirely refractory to benzodiazepines.

   (a) In adults, treat initially with midazolam 10 mg IM, or lorazepam 4 mg IV, or diazepam 10 mg IV.

   (b) In children (2–12 years or 13–40 kg), treat initially with either fixed or weight-based doses. Use weight-based doses for infants, and either weight-based or the same fixed doses used in adult dosing for teenagers. Treat with midazolam 5 mg IM, or lorazepam 2 mg (or 0.1 mg/kg) IV, or diazepam 5 mg (or 0.2 mg/kg) IV.

   (c) In both adults and children, repeat the initial dose 10 minutes after administration if convulsions persist.

3. *In adults, intravenous diazepam appears (but is not proven) to be less effective than intravenous lorazepam at stopping seizures in the prehospital setting.*

Studies

The PHTSE trial suggested, but did not have the statistical power to prove, that IV lorazepam is more effective than IV diazepam in the prehospital treatment of status epilepticus. However, randomized controlled data from other similar settings is corroborative of these findings. In the landmark VA Cooperative study of 199 patients treated in the hospital, efficacy was 67 percent with IV lorazepam and 60 percent in the group whose treatment included IV diazepam.[28] Similar or greater effect differences were identified by others.[5, 6, 29, 30] The best available data (moderate quality) suggests that diazepam (by any route) should be replaced by more effective benzodiazepines like lorazepam or midazolam.

4. *Intranasal and buccal midazolam appear (but are not proven) to be equally or more effective than intravenous or rectal diazepam at stopping seizures.*

Studies

Diazepam is often administered rectally to seizing patients, both by caregivers of patients with epilepsy and in some EMS systems, but efficacy has not been well established in status epilepticus.[6, 31] Most controlled data on the use of rectal diazepam has been generated by trials of patients with repetitive (rather than continuous) seizures, and most have been performed in settings outside of North America. Among 98 children with status epilepticus treated in Tehran and randomly assigned to rectal diazepam or buccal midazolam, 82 percent were controlled with rectal diazepam at 5 minutes as compared to 100 percent of those treated with buccal midazolam.[32] Results, however, vary dramatically from study to study. In 2005, an open label, quasi-randomized (alternating) trial of 219 children in pediatric emergency departments with any seizure found efficacy at 10 minutes in 41 percent of those receiving rectal diazepam, compared to 65 percent in another group treated with buccal midazolam.[11] Other, much smaller, trials have found rectal diazepam to be more effective, but have also confirmed the efficacy of buccal midazolam. An open label, quasi-randomized (alternating) study of buccal midazolam versus rectal diazepam in 22 patients in a residential epilepsy center found efficacy to be 74 vs. 83 percent at 2 hours.[13] Despite the heterogeneity of these studies and their small sample sizes, the best available data suggest that non-intravenous routes of midazolam are consistently as good as or markedly superior to rectal diazepam.[12]

As noted earlier, the PHTSE and RAMPART trials taken together provide high quality evidence that IM midazolam is superior to IV lorazepam and by inference IV diazepam, but how do the other non-intravenous routes (buccal and nasal, mostly) of midazolam compare to IV diazepam? Buccal and nasal administration appear to have pharmacodynamics and pharmacokinetics similar to IM administration of midazolam, so they might be expected to work as well as the IM route provided the medicine is not blown or spat out by the convulsing patient. Again, specific data are limited. In 92 children, seizure termination by 10 minutes was 69 percent with buccal midazolam and

70 percent in those with intravenous diazepam.[33] A meta-analysis of prior small trials also found similar efficacy between all non-IV routes and IV diazepam.[12] Although there are no high quality data, the best available information suggests that buccal or nasal administration of midazolam, in appropriate doses, are reasonable alternatives to intravenous diazepam.

Low-quality recommendations

1. *Because the best supportive care during status epilepticus is to stop the seizure, definitive therapy with benzodiazepines should generally precede other interventions.* Generalized tonic–clonic seizures can cause respiratory depression, aspiration and hemodynamic compromise, especially when convulsions go on for a long time. Supportive measures in patients with prolonged convulsions are appropriate as required. It should be noted, however, that rapid termination of convulsive seizures is generally more effective than supportive measures in treating the respiratory and cardiovascular complications of status epilepticus. In most circumstances, definitive treatment for seizures with benzodiazepines should precede measures such as intravenous therapy and endotracheal intubation.

2. Because the physiologic manifestations of the post-ictal period are generally transient and benign, most patients without other underlying problems can be managed with observation immediately after cessation of seizures.

The period after termination of seizures is typically characterized by a diminished level of consciousness both as a consequence of the post-ictal state itself and from the sedating effects of benzodiazepine therapy. Although airway reflexes may be diminished, and there may be some respiratory and cardiovascular depression, the post-ictal state is most often transient and can be best managed by observation alone or brief temporizing interventions (repositioning of the head and neck or body position, or use of an oral or nasopharangeal airway). More definitive (and invasive) methods of support including endotracheal intubation should still be used when required, but this is uncommon and is usually the consequence of an underlying pathology that caused the seizure (like an intracranial bleed, for example).

3. *Patients with prolonged seizure symptoms without awakening that are suspected to be "pseudo-seizure" should usually be treated with benzodiazepines in the same manner as any other seizure patient.* Pseudo-seizures are psychogenic, non-epileptic spells that can mimic status epilepticus. Although the most obvious manifestations of this can reasonably be diagnosed in the prehospital setting and treated as a primary psychiatric emergency, such presentations are relatively rare. More often, certainty in differentiating suspected pseudo-seizure from epileptic convulsions requires substantial expertise and may require diagnostic EEG testing. Diagnosis is often complicated because many patients with pseudo-seizures also have a

history of true epileptic seizures. Ultimately, the potential danger to the patient of delaying benzodiazepines in status epilepticus is great, while benzodiazepines are relatively safe (and can even be effective) in patients with pseudo-seizure.

Summary

Seizures are a common cause of EMS activation. Single, uncomplicated and self-limited seizures in patients with a known seizure disorder are the most frequent presentations. Such patients require little prehospital care and may not require transportation. Persistent or rapidly recurring seizures are a life-threatening medical emergency. Rapid administration of adequate doses of benzodiazepines is effective at stopping convulsion prior to ED arrival and decreasing the likelihood of both hospital and ICU admission. The best available data suggest that intramuscular midazolam is the most effective route and agent in the prehospital setting. Prehospital treatment also involves supportive care during both the convulsions and the post-ictal state. Prehospital care should also involve a very brief evaluation of potentially life-threatening causes of seizure that can be treated during EMS care, such as hypoglycemia, arrhythmia or acute injury. Pyschogenic, non-epileptic spells (psuedo-seizures) are often challenging to diagnose in any setting and should generally be an EMS diagnosis in only the most extreme and obvious presentation.

Key issues for future investigation

Can family members safely provide more effective benzodiazepine therapy through more optimal non-IV dosing prior to EMS arrival? Patients with epilepsy are often prescribed a form of diazepam for family members to administer rectally to the patient in case of rapidly recurrent or persistent seizures, but rectal diazepam is frequently not administered for a variety of reasons, and when it is, it has limited bioavailability and efficacy. Intramuscular autoinjectors or intranasal atomizers of midazolam may be more effective at terminating seizures prior to EMS arrival, if they can be used safely in this scenario.

Can a clinical decision rule or guideline be developed to safely identify (or risk stratify) those seizure patients evaluated by EMS who can be safely managed without transport and ED evaluation? Many patients with breakthrough seizures do not require diagnostic or therapeutic management by EMS or in the ED, but there are no proven criteria or guidelines to assist either patients or EMS providers in reliably distinguishing episodes that do require emergency care from those that do not. Such a decision aid could be developed from observational data sets and would then be optimally evaluated prospectively in a clinical study.

Can the efficacy of prehospital therapy for status epilepticus be improved by simultaneous treatment with both early adequate benzodiazepine dosing and earlier rapid administration of a "second-line" anticonvulsant agent? Traditionally, second-line anticonvulsant agents that operate at non-GABAergic sites of action have been given in patients with status epilepticus only in the emergency department after the patient failed to respond to benzodiazepines. Most second-line agents require slow, controlled, intravenous infusions and are therefore not very well suited to delivery in the field, but at least one existing agent, fosphenytoin, and some newer agents under development, can be given in a single rapid dose, preferably intramuscularly. Accelerating treatment of SE by giving first- and second-line agents in parallel rather than serially could have two possible benefits. It could reduce the number of refractory cases by giving the second-line agents at a time they are more likely to be effective. It could also improve outcomes by allowing more rapid identification of the patients with truly refractory SE, which would permit advancing to definitive therapy with general anesthesia much earlier in the patient's course. This interesting idea, however, remains entirely speculative at this time.

REFERENCES

1. Alldredge, B. K., Gelb, A. M., Isaacs, S. M. *et al.* (2001). "A comparison of lorazepam, diazepam, and placebo for the treatment of out-of-hospital status epilepticus," *N. Engl. J. Med.* 345(9): 631–7.
2. Lowenstein, D. H., Bleck, T. and Macdonald, R. L. (1999). "It's time to revise the definition of status epilepticus," *Epilepsia* 40(1): 120–2.

3. Silbergleit, R., Durkalski, V., Lowenstein, D. *et al.* (2012). "Intramuscular versus intravenous therapy for prehospital status epilepticus," *N. Engl. J. Med.* 366(7): 591–600.

4. Millikan, D., Rice, B. and Silbergleit, R. (2009). "Emergency treatment of status epilepticus: current thinking," *Emerg. Med. Clin. North Am.* 27(1): 101–13, ix.

5. Food and Drug Administration (1997). "NDA approval package 18140/S003," available at www.fda.gov.

6. Appleton, R., Sweeney, A., Choonara, I. *et al.* (1995). "Lorazepam versus diazepam in the acute treatment of epileptic seizures and status epilepticus," *Dev. Med. Child Neurol.* 37(8): 682–8.

7. Brophy, G. M., Bell, R., Claassen, J. *et al.* (2012). "Guidelines for the evaluation and management of status epilepticus," *Neurocrit. Care* 17(1): 3–23.

8. Cock, H. R. and Schapira, A. H. (2002). "A comparison of lorazepam and diazepam as initial therapy in convulsive status epilepticus," *QJM* 95(4): 225–31.

9. Claassen, J., Silbergleit, R., Weingart, S. D. *et al.* (2012). "Emergency neurological life support: status epilepticus," *Neurocrit. Care* 17(Suppl. 1): S73–8.

10. Alfonzo-Echeverri, E., Troutman, K. C. and George, W. (1990). "Absorption and elimination of midazolam by submucosal and intramuscular routes," *Anesth. Prog.* 37(6): 277–81.

11. McIntyre, J., Robertson, S., Norris, E. *et al.* (2005). "Safety and efficacy of buccal midazolam versus rectal diazepam for emergency treatment of seizures in children: a randomised controlled trial," *Lancet* 366(9481): 205–10.

12. McMullan, J., Sasson, C., Pancioli, A. *et al.* (2010). "Midazolam versus diazepam for the treatment of status epilepticus in children and young adults: a meta-analysis," *Acad. Emerg. Med.* 17(6): 575–82.

13. Nakken, K. O. and Lossius, M. I. (2011). "Buccal midazolam or rectal diazepam for treatment of residential adult patients with serial seizures or status epilepticus," *Acta Neurol. Scand.* 124(2): 99–103.

14. Siket, M. S. and Merchant, R. C. (2011). "Psychogenic seizures: a review and description of pitfalls in their acute diagnosis and management in the emergency department," *Emerg. Med. Clin. North Am.* 29(1): 73–81.

15. Martindale, J. L., Goldstein, J. N. and Pallin, D. J. (2011). "Emergency department seizure epidemiology," *Emerg. Med. Clin. North Am.* 29(1): 15–27.

16. French, J. A., Kanner, A. M., Bautista, J. *et al.* (2004). "Efficacy and tolerability of the new antiepileptic drugs I: treatment of new onset epilepsy: report of the Therapeutics and Technology Assessment Subcommittee and Quality Standards Subcommittee of the American Academy of Neurology and the American Epilepsy Society," *Neurology* 62(8): 1252–60.

17. Bassin, S., Smith, T. L. and Bleck, T. P. (2002). "Clinical review: status epilepticus," *Crit. Care* 6(2): 137–42.

18. Claassen, J., Lokin, J. K., Fitzsimmons, B. F. *et al.* (2002). "Predictors of functional disability and mortality after status epilepticus," *Neurology* 58(1): 139–42.

19. DeLorenzo, R. J., Hauser, W. A., Towne, A. R. *et al.* (1996). "A prospective, population-based epidemiologic study

of status epilepticus in Richmond, Virginia," *Neurology* 46(4): 1029–35.

20. Penberthy, L. T., Towne, A., Garnett, L. K. *et al.* (2005). "Estimating the economic burden of status epilepticus to the health care system," *Seizure* 14(1): 46–51.

21. Wu, Y. W., Shek, D. W., Garcia, P. A. *et al.* (2002). "Incidence and mortality of generalized convulsive status epilepticus in California," *Neurology* 58(7): 1070–6.

22. Maillard, L., Jonas, J., Boyer, R. *et al.* (2012). "One-year outcome after a first clinically possible epileptic seizure: predictive value of clinical classification and early EEG," *Neurophysiol. Clin.* 42(6): 355–62.

23. Sierra-Marcos, A., Toledo, M., Quintana, M. *et al.* (2011). "Diagnosis of epileptic syndrome after a new onset seizure and its correlation at long-term follow-up: longitudinal study of 131 patients from the emergency room," *Epilepsy Res.* 97(1–2): 30–6.

24. Fujikawa, D. (2006). "The two faces of electrographic status epilepticus: the walking wounded and the ictally comatose" in C. Wasterlain and D. Treiman (eds.), *Status Epilepticus: Mechanisms and Management* (Cambridge: MIT Press), pp. 109–12.

25. Lowenstein, D. H., Alldredge, B. K., Allen, F. *et al.* (2001). "The prehospital treatment of status epilepticus (PHTSE) study: design and methodology," *Control Clin. Trials* 22(3): 290–309.

26. McMullan, J. T., Pinnawin, A., Jones, E. *et al.* (2013). "The 60-day temperature-dependent degradation of midazolam

and Lorazepam in the prehospital environment," *Prehosp. Emerg. Care* 17(1): 1–7.

27. Chamberlain, J. (2008). "Efficacy and safety study comparing lorazepam and diazepam for children in the emergency department with seizures" (National Institutes of Health), available at http://clinicaltrials.gov/ct2/show/ NCT00621478.

28. Treiman, D. M., Meyers, P. D., Walton, N. Y. *et al.* (1998). "A comparison of four treatments for generalized convulsive status epilepticus. Veterans Affairs Status Epilepticus Cooperative Study Group," *N. Engl. J. Med.* 339(12): 792–8.

29. Giang, D. W. and McBride, M. C. (1988). "Lorazepam versus diazepam for the treatment of status epilepticus," *Pediatr. Neurol.* 4(6): 358–61.

30. Leppik, I. E., Derivan, A. T., Homan, R. W. *et al.* (1983). "Double-blind study of lorazepam and diazepam in status epilepticus," *JAMA* 249(11): 1452–4.

31. Cereghino, J. J., Cloyd, J. C. and Kuzniecky, R. I. (2002). "Rectal diazepam gel for treatment of acute repetitive seizures in adults," *Arch. Neurol.* 59(12): 1915–20.

32. Ashrafi, M. R., Khosroshahi, N., Karimi, P. *et al.* (2010). "Efficacy and usability of buccal midazolam in controlling acute prolonged convulsive seizures in children," *Eur. J. Paediatr. Neurol.* 14(5): 434–8.

33. Tonekaboni, S. H., Shamsabadi, F. M., Anvari, S. S. *et al.* (2012). "A comparison of buccal midazolam and intravenous diazepam for the acute treatment of seizures in children," *Iran J. Pediatr.* 22(3): 303–8.

Chapter 4

Stroke and transient ischemic attack

Stephanie A. Crapo, John M. Wooten, and Jane H. Brice

Recommendations (Table 4.1)

High quality

1. Testing glucose levels is critical. Glucose levels less than 60 mg/dL should be treated in the prehospital setting.
2. Rapid delivery of acute stroke patients to stroke centers capable of providing state-of-the-art stroke care is imperative. To achieve this goal, EMS systems should establish firm transport guidelines for providers as a part of stroke protocols that enable EMS providers to transport acute stroke patients to appropriate facilities.
3. EMS providers should prenotify receiving facilities of the impending arrival of an acute stroke patient as soon as possible.

Moderate quality

1. 9-1-1 centers should utilize a validated algorithm for stroke recognition during a call for medical assistance.

Prehospital Care of Neurologic Emergencies, ed. Todd J. Crocco and Michael R. Sayre. Published by Cambridge University Press. © Cambridge University Press 2014.

Table 4.1 Recommendations and level of evidence

CVA/TIA level of recommendation table

Class I: Procedure/treatment should be performed/administered	Class IIa: It is reasonable to perform procedure/administer treatment	Class IIb: Procedure/treatment may be considered	Class III: Treatment/procedure provides no benefit and should not be considered
EMS providers should use a standardized stroke scale.	The LAPSS can be effective at ruling out stroke mimics.	The usefulness of managing hypertension in the prehospital setting is not proven.	Oxygen should not be administered to patients without signs of hypoxia.
EMS providers should measure the blood glucose of all patients with suspected stroke and treat hypoglycemia.	All hospitals should have stroke treatment plans in place, and share this information with EMS.	The effectiveness of induced hypothermia is not known.	Use of neuroprotective agents is not recommended.
EMS should transport stroke patients to a dedicated stroke facility when it is within a reasonable distance.		EMS systems may consider setting a target on-scene time for patients with suspected acute stroke.	
EMS providers should prenotify receiving facilities of the impending arrival of an acute stroke patient as soon as possible.		9-1-1 centers may consider use of a validated stroke algorithm.	

2. EMS systems should utilize a validated stroke scale in their service and train all providers in the appropriate use of the scale. EMS providers should utilize the scale on all suspected stroke patients and document the results.

3. Utilize supplemental oxygen to maintain oxygen saturation greater than 94 percent. Supplemental oxygen is not recommended in patients without hypoxia.

Low quality

1. In order to reduce on-scene times and improve onset-to-treatment times, EMS systems should set a target on-scene time for patients with suspected acute stroke.

2. The benefit of routine prehospital management of hypertension is not proven. If intervention is necessary, it should be done in conjunction with medical control.

3. Benefit of induced hypothermia is not proven. No neuroprotective agent has proven efficacy, and use of neuroprotective agents is not recommended.

Overview

Stroke is a medical emergency for which Emergency Medical Services (EMS) plays a critical role in identification and timely transport to an appropriate receiving facility. A stroke occurs when brain tissue dies secondary to insufficient blood supply.[1] The reason for insufficient brain blood supply can be divided into two broad categories: 1. interruption of supply secondary to clot or embolus (ischemic stroke); and 2. supply interruption due to rupture of the vascular supply (hemorrhagic stroke). The vast majority of strokes are ischemic, with over 85 percent of strokes being caused by a blockage of a blood vessel in the brain or neck, and the remainder falling into the hemorrhagic category.[1]

When all the pieces fall into place, stroke patients may be eligible for brain-saving therapy and treatment with a promising survival and recovery rate.[2] Stroke represents the fourth leading cause of death in the United States, with approximately 130,000 deaths due to stroke each year.[3] On average, an American has a stroke every 40 seconds and dies from stroke every 4 minutes.[4] Mortality, however, represents the tip of the stroke burden in the United States. Every year, approximately 795,000 Americans have a stroke, making it a leading cause of serious long-term disability.[4] Stroke also represents a huge financial burden. Including the cost of health services, medications and missed days of work, the financial burden of stroke is estimated to be $53.9 billion each year in the United States.[5]

Approximately 15 percent of all strokes are preceded by a transient ischemic attack (TIA).[6] Persons having a TIA have an increased risk for subsequently having a stroke. In a recent study of 1,707 TIA patients, 11 percent experienced a subsequent stroke within 90 days and 5 percent had a stroke within 2 days.[7] In a paper combining several studies into one analysis, the short-term risk of stroke after TIA was found to be between 3 and 10 percent at 2 days and 9 and 17 percent at 90 days.[8, 9] Thus, it is critical for EMS providers to recognize stroke-like symptoms and respond in an evidence-based manner utilizing the most current guidelines and protocols.

Despite representing approximately 2.7 percent of 9-1-1 calls for EMS service, stroke is a time-critical illness for which EMS services make a difference in outcome.[10] Treatment for acute ischemic stroke requires rapid recognition of symptoms and prompt arrival at an emergency department prepared to deliver thrombolytic therapy or other advanced care. Thrombolytic therapy must be delivered within 4.5 hours from the time the patient was last seen neurologically at baseline to be effective.[2] In a Californian study, 23.5 percent of stroke patients arrived in the emergency department within 3 hours of stroke onset and 4.3 percent met criteria for thrombolytic administration.[11] The study authors calculated that if all of the EMS stroke patients had called 9-1-1 immediately upon onset of symptoms, an estimated 28.6 percent of patients would have received thrombolytic therapy and if all the stroke patients had recognized symptoms and called 9-1-1 immediately, 57 percent could have received thrombolytic treatment.[11]

We present a set of key challenges and recommendations for the prehospital care of stroke. The EMS care of a stroke patient is critical and important elements in delivery of this brain-saving care include: the role of EMS dispatch; EMS recognition and intervention; prenotification of the receiving hospital; and destination decision making to deliver the right patient to the right facility in the right amount of time.

Key challenges

Stroke recognition

Dispatch

In almost all studies of delay in stroke care, the 9-1-1 call has been shown to be the most critical factor predicting emergency department arrival within the time window for intervention therapy.[12] Despite the significant role of the 9-1-1 center in the delivery of stroke care, few studies have assessed the ability of the 9-1-1 telecommunicator to use assessment algorithms to recognize stroke during a 9-1-1 call. We know that without assessment algorithms, 9-1-1 telecommunicators recognize stroke poorly. As an example, in a North Carolina study of 93 EMS patients with hospital-confirmed stroke, 45 percent of callers mentioned stroke in the 9-1-1 call, but only 31 percent of the calls were dispatched as a stroke and 31 percent as sick calls.[13] It is estimated that, nationally, 9-1-1 telecommunicators recognize stroke less that 50 percent of the time during a 9-1-1 call.[12]

Several investigators have begun to assess whether or not 9-1-1 recognition of stroke increases when an assessment algorithm is used during the 9-1-1 call. Liferidge examined the ability of laypersons to receive stroke assessment instructions during a mock 9-1-1 call and to accurately perform an assessment.[14] Hurwitz took that one step further and evaluated whether laypersons could accurately relay neurological deficits to a 9-1-1 telecommunicator.[15] They found that laypersons can: 1. understand directions to perform a structured neurological assessment based on the Cincinnati

Prehospital Stroke Scale; 2. perform the assessment accurately; and 3. relay those findings correctly to a telecommunicator. These studies formed the basis for structured stroke assessment algorithms currently in use in validated 9-1-1 protocols. Ramanujam found that use of the Medical Priority Dispatch System stroke algorithm resulted in a 9-1-1 telecommunicator sensitivity of 83 percent and a positive predictive value of 42 percent. This means that when a telecommunicator classifies a call as a stroke, they are right approximately 42 percent of the time; however, it also means that they cast a wide net and miss only about 17 percent of true strokes.[16] Finally, a German team has developed a new algorithm for 9-1-1 detection of stroke. Their tool assesses for "sudden new" neurological symptoms or a unilateral face droop or arm weakness or speech difficulty. In a trial of the new assessment tool, 9-1-1 telecommunicators correctly identified 59 percent of all true strokes. The assessment tool warrants further investigation.[17]

EMS providers

While EMS providers play an integral role in reducing the window of time from symptom onset to treatment initiation, they must first accurately recognize stroke during their patient assessment in order to initiate the cascade of events required to begin therapy. A 2008 study has shown that improving the ability of EMS providers to identify stroke using screening tools can increase thrombolytic therapy rates by as much as 21 percent.[18] In order to accurately and consistently identify prehospital patients with acute stroke, several stroke scales have been created.

Most available prehospital stroke scales derive from the National Institutes of Health (NIH) stroke scale.[19] This comprehensive 15-item stroke assessment was originally designed for use in clinical trials.[20] Having proved effective in discriminating stroke severity, it is now used in general practice to grade stroke severity and to evaluate patients for thrombolytic therapy.[21] Unfortunately for prehospital providers, the scale takes up to 8 minutes to complete even in skilled and practiced hands.[20] In the time-dependent prehospital environment, 8 minutes is much too long for an assessment tool. Among the first to recognize the need for a brief prehospital assessment tool were investigators from the University of Cincinnati.

Kothari *et al.* in developing the Cincinnati Prehospital Stroke Scale (CPSS) used three of the NIH scale elements – facial weakness, arm weakness and speech difficulty – which allowed physicians to discriminate stroke with 92 percent specificity.[22] The CPSS in use today asks EMS personnel to evaluate patients on three elements: facial droop during smiling, arm drift with eyes closed, and repetition of a sentence to assess speech as normal or abnormal (Table 4.2). If any one of the assessments is judged to be abnormal, then the scale is considered to be positive for stroke. The CPSS has been studied in a variety of settings. Kothari *et al.* studied EMS performance as compared to physicians in an inpatient stroke population, finding the sensitivity of the scale to be 66 percent for physicians and 59 percent for EMS personnel, with a specificity of 87 and 89 percent, respectively.[23] The sensitivity of a test or assessment tool represents the ability of the test not

Table 4.2 Cincinnati Prehospital Stroke Scale (CPSS)

A. Facial droop

1. Normal: Both sides of face move equally
2. Abnormal: One side of face does not move at all

B. Arm drift

1. Normal: Both arms move equally or not at all
2. Abnormal: One arm drifts compared to the other

C. Speech

1. Normal: Patient uses correct words with no slurring
2. Abnormal: Slurred or inappropriate words or no speech at all

Source: Kothari *et al.* 1999.

to miss strokes and the specificity represents the ability to not assign a diagnosis of stroke when the patient really does not have a stroke. In other words, the higher the sensitivity, the fewer missed strokes; the higher the specificity, the fewer stroke mimics detected. He also found that the CPSS poorly identifies patients with posterior circulation strokes who often present with dizziness or poor balance as their predominant symptoms.[23]

More recently, CPSS has been tested in actual practice in the prehospital environment. Ramanujam *et al.* conducted a retrospective study of paramedic assessment for 477 stroke patients in Southern California, finding a sensitivity of 44 percent and a positive predictive value of 40 percent for paramedics using the CPSS.[16] Frendl *et al.* studied CPSS use in Durham, North Carolina after a 1-hour educational intervention. Of 154 patients with suspected stroke, 61 had a final diagnosis of stroke, leading to a sensitivity of 71 percent and specificity of 52 percent.[24] The CPSS sensitivity and specificity in actual field practice appears to be lower than that found in an inpatient setting.

Kidwell *et al.* developed a prehospital stroke evaluation tool that was designed to reduce the number of stroke mimics included in prehospital stroke alerts. The Los Angeles Prehospital Stroke Screen (LAPSS) includes patient history, blood glucose measurement and motor deficits in the assessment algorithm (see Table 4.3).[25] When used retrospectively in patients enrolled in a stroke trial, the sensitivity was 92 percent and the specificity was 93 percent. In field use of the LAPSS in Los Angeles, the sensitivity of the scale was 91 percent and the specificity 99 percent, with a positive predictive value of 97 percent and accuracy of 98 percent.[26] A more recent German study found a sensitivity of 68.3 percent and a specificity of 85.1 percent.[27]

Several other stroke scales have been developed, but none demonstrate better test parameters than the LAPSS. Studnek *et al.* attempted to develop a new stroke scale, Med PACS, which integrated elements from the CPSS and the LAPSS together with locally derived elements. In their study, the CPSS demonstrated a sensitivity of 79 percent and a specificity of 24 percent. The Med PACS did little better, with a sensitivity of 74 percent and a specificity of 33 percent.[28] By modifying the CPSS slightly, Japanese investigators are testing the ability of their test, the Maria Prehospital Stroke Scale (MPSS), to predict the need for thrombolytic therapy after

Table 4.3 Los Angeles Prehospital Stroke Screen (LAPSS)

Screening criteria

	Yes	No
1. Age over 45 years	—	—
2. No prior history of seizure disorder	—	—
3. New onset of neurological symptoms in last 24 hours	—	—
4. Patient was ambulatory at baseline (prior to event)	—	—
5. Blood glucose between 60 and 400	—	

Exam criteria

	Normal	Right	Left
Facial smile/grimace	—	— Droop	— Droop
Grip	—	— Weak grip — No grip	— Weak grip — No grip
Arm weakness	—	— Drifts down — Falls rapidly	— Drifts down — Falls rapidly

	Yes	No
6. Based on exam, patient has only unilateral weakness	—	—

If **YES** (or unknown) to all items above, LAPSS screening criteria met.

If LAPSS criteria for stroke met, call receiving hospital with "code stroke."

Source: Kidwell *et al.* 2000.

transportation.[29] The MPSS assesses the three CPSS physical examination findings, but grades them differently. Facial droop is graded as normal (0) or abnormal (1), and the other two items are graded in three levels as normal (0), not severe (1) and severe (2). As the MPSS increased in value, the rate of thrombolytic therapy also increased from 0 percent for a score of 0 up to 31.5 percent for a maximum score of 5. It is important to note that the MPSS is designed to predict the need for thrombolytic therapy rather than to determine a potential diagnosis of stroke.[29]

The ROSIER (Recognition of Stroke in the Emergency Room) was developed by investigators in the United Kingdom for use by emergency physicians working in an emergency department.[30] Chinese researchers have extended the use of the scale to the prehospital setting, although again for use by emergency physicians who staff their EMS response vehicles.[31] The ROSIER assesses elements of history (no seizure, no syncope, recent onset of symptoms) and physical examination (asymmetrical facial, arm or leg weakness, speech disturbance and visual field deficits) to produce a score between 2 and 5. Patients with a total score of >0 are taken as being consistent with stroke, whereas scores of 0 signify a low probability of stroke. When used by emergency physicians in a prehospital setting, the ROSIER showed a sensitivity of 89.97 percent and a specificity of 83.23 percent.[31] Use of the ROSIER by prehospital providers is still to be studied.

The Melbourne Ambulance Stroke Screen (MASS) was developed by Janet Bray and colleagues in Australia.[32] The MASS was created in an attempt to combine the strengths of the CPSS and the LAPSS. The CPSS has been found to have a higher sensitivity in detecting stroke and the LAPSS to have a higher specificity. By combining elements from both scales, Dr. Bray hoped to create a tool with both high sensitivity and specificity. The MASS asks EMS personnel to determine the answers to history questions (age >45, no seizure, ambulatory at baseline and normal blood glucose), as well as physical examination assessments (unilateral facial droop, grip weakness or arm drift and abnormal speech). To be considered a stroke, all of the history questions must be answered affirmatively and at least one physical examination abnormality must be present.[32] In her initial study, MASS was compared to CPSS and LAPSS in field use by 18 paramedics. The MASS showed a sensitivity of 90 percent (CPSS 95 percent, LAPSS 78 percent) and a specificity of 74 percent (CPSS 56 percent, LAPSS 85 percent).[32] In a subsequent test, Bray et al. studied the use of MASS as compared to CPSS in field practice over a five-month period. MASS sensitivity was 83 percent as compared to CPSS sensitivity of 88 percent, and the specificity was 86 percent for MASS and 79 percent for CPSS.[33]

The FAST test (Face, Arm, Speech, Time) developed in the United Kingdom asks prehospital providers to evaluate for facial droop, arm weakness and speech difficulty. If any one of the three is positive, then they are asked to notify the receiving hospital in a timely fashion.[34] Two evaluations of the FAST test have been published. Harbison et al. in 2003 reported 79 percent accuracy for paramedics using the tool.[34] Nor et al. reported 78 percent accuracy with very good agreement between paramedic assessments and neurologist evaluations.[35]

Lacombe *et al.* first reported development of the Miami Emergency Neurologic Deficit (MEND) Examination in 2000.[36] This 12-item tool incorporates all three components of the Cincinnati Prehospital Stroke Scale (CPSS) and six additional components from the NIHSS. In actual use, the MEND was found to have 78 percent accuracy.[37] Investigators in Ontario have developed a tool very similar to the CPSS.[38] The Ontario Prehospital Stroke Screening Tool comprises three physical examination assessments (unilateral weakness, slurred speech or muteness, and facial droop), combined with a 2-hour time limit from symptom onset, and six exclusion criteria (hypoglycemia, seizure, critically ill, resolved symptoms, Glasgow Coma Score less than 10, and terminally ill or palliative care patients). When the Ontario Stroke Screening Tool returned a positive result in the field, it was correct 89.5 percent of the time.[38]

None of the stroke scales available to the prehospital provider are perfect. They each have their strengths and weaknesses. Most err on the side of "over-triage" of possible stroke patients to avoid missing acute strokes. What seems to be most important is that EMS providers utilize a validated stroke scale in their field assessments of potential stroke patients.

Treatment

Treatment of a stroke begins prehospital in several key areas, including glucose testing and management, hypertension, oxygen therapy and neuroprotectives. In an ischemic stroke, the area surrounding the ischemic tissue has been labeled the ischemic penumbra. These cells are not yet ischemic and often lie in a dormant state. They are at a higher risk of injury if the ischemic insult is extended, such as with hypoglycemia, hypertension, hypotension or hypoxia.

Hypoglycemia

Hypoglycemia is a well-known stroke mimic. Neurologic symptoms of hypoglycemia vary, but include psychomotor abnormalities including hemiparesis, impaired cognition and, at severe levels, can include seizure and coma.[39] Multiple case reports exist that show presentations of hypoglycemia as hemiplegia (typically right-sided and associated with slurred speech). The symptoms, if caused by hypoglycemia, fully resolve after administration of glucose, many times obviating the need for cerebrovascular evaluation.[40–2] One study undertaken by Megarbane looked at 25 patients with intentional insulin overdose to investigate prognostic factors in insulin poisoning. The results indicate that hypoglycemia duration rather than depth results in poor clinical outcome.[43] *It is therefore critical to test the glucose level prehospital and treat if the level is below 60 mg/dL with a goal of normoglycemia.*[44]

Blood pressure

Hypertension is a known risk factor for developing a stroke, and elevated blood pressure is observed in over 80 percent of patients following an ischemic stroke.[45] It is not known, however, whether this rise in blood pressure is due to a protective sympathetic response to the stroke, pre-existing hypertension, loss of autoregulation or the pathology of the stroke itself. The perfusion of the brain, or cerebral perfusion pressure (CPP), is related to the mean arterial pressure (MAP) minus the intracranial pressure (ICP) (CPP = MAP – ICP). It is theorized that the perfusion distal to the occluded vessel in a stroke is low, causing dilation of the vessels. The perfusion of the tissue distal to the obstruction is therefore dependent upon the systemic blood pressure.[46, 47] This is the pathophysiologic basis behind permissive hypertension in acute stroke, or allowing systemic hypertension to continue in order to preserve CPP. However, excessive hypertension can have deleterious effects such as cerebral edema.[48] In-hospital in the acute setting, treatment is typically reserved for systolic pressure greater than 220 mmHg or diastolic pressure greater than 120 mmHg except when treating with reperfusion therapy when tighter control of blood pressure is required.[49] Data to support prehospital management of hypertension are lacking, and the recommendations are extrapolated from in-hospital studies.

High or low blood pressure is associated with worse outcomes in acute stroke. Vemmos *et al.* found a U-shaped relationship between admission blood pressure and mortality, with the U point at SBP 130 mmHg.[50] Their prospective study examined 1,121 patients admitted to a university hospital in Greece with a stroke within 24 hours of onset and followed up for 12 months. They measured mortality at 1 and 12 months in relation to admission systolic and diastolic blood pressures. Low admission blood pressure-values were associated with patients with congestive heart failure and coronary artery disease, and death tended to be due to cardiovascular disease. Stead *et al.* also found increased mortality among stroke patients exhibiting low systolic blood pressures in the first 24 hours after stroke.[51] High admission blood pressure-values were associated with pre-existing hypertension and with lacunar infarcts. Their deaths tended to be due to cerebral edema. In a review, Wilmot *et al.* found that high blood pressure in acute stroke is associated with death, dependency and deterioration.[52] However, acutely lowering blood pressure may be detrimental. A study undertaken by Oliveira-Filho *et al.* in Bahia, Brazil found that blood pressure reduction in the first 24 hours following stroke onset is independently associated with poor outcomes at 3 months. They studied 115 consecutive patients admitted within 24 hours following stroke onset. Among other factors noted, a larger degree of systolic blood pressure reduction was independently associated with poor outcomes at 3 months.[53]

Hypertension in acute stroke is a delicate balance. Deleterious effects are seen with blood pressures too high as well as with lowering the blood pressures. Small changes in systemic blood pressure can have a large impact on cerebral perfusion. Thus, in the prehospital setting, routine management of hypertension is not recommended except in prolonged transport times and when transporting between stroke centers. This should be done in conjunction with medical control.[54, 55]

Hypoxemia

Oxygen is a powerful medication that can be used to treat hypoxemia. Following a stroke, stroke victims are at risk from hypoxemia due to aspiration, hypoventilation and upper airway obstruction.[44] Ronning and Guldvog in Norway conducted a quasi-randomized study to evaluate the use of oxygen in stroke patients. Patients who were admitted within 24 hours of stroke onset were distributed into the study group that received oxygen therapy at 3L/min. or the control group who did not receive supplemental oxygen. Main outcomes measured were one-year survival, disability 7 months after the stroke, and neurological impairment. They found that the oxygen-supplemented group trended toward mortality and concluded that oxygen should not be used routinely in stroke treatment.[56] Use of oxygen when there is no evidence of hypoxemia can cause hyperoxia, which also has untoward effects. Hyperoxia is associated with cerebral vasoconstriction, as well as increased oxygen free radicals. These can increase the ischemic injury in stroke.[57, 58] *Presently, oxygen should be used to treat hypoxemia and titrated to prevent hyperoxia.*[59]

Neuroprotectives

There are two categories of treatment of acute stroke. One is improving the blood flow as with use of thrombolytics and antiplatelet agents. The other is targeting the molecular pathophysiology of ischemic injury such as with neuroprotective agents.[60] Neuroprotectives are an exciting area of research, and some of the investigated agents include albumin, alcohol plus caffeine, anti-inflammatory medications, free-radical scavengers, calcium channel blockers, sodium channel blockers, glutamate antagonists, nitric oxide inhibitors, statins and more.[49, 60] Some of these agents have shown great promise in animal models of stroke, but no agent has proven effective in phase III clinical trials in humans. For example, nimodipine, a calcium channel blocker, is used after subarachnoid hemorrhage to dilate cerebral vessels and prevent vasospasm with very little effect on systemic blood pressure. In theory, if the same pathophysiologic principles apply in stroke, nimodipine could help restore blood flow distal to the obstruction and improve stroke outcomes. In the VENUS trial, study participants were randomized into oral nimodipine versus placebo and were treated within 6 hours of stroke onset for a duration of 10 days. No difference in outcomes between the study groups was found.[61] *More research is needed to find a neuroprotective agent that has proven efficacy in human models. As such, neuroprotectives are not currently recommended for use in the prehospital setting.*[49]

Scene management

EMS scene management in setting of acute CVA

With the advent of thrombolytic therapy for acute ischemic stroke, reducing the time from the onset of symptoms to definitive medical care is crucial to improving patient outcomes. The current guidelines recommended by the American Stroke Association set a target treatment window of 3 hours from symptom onset.[49] Many studies have examined the common causes in delay of treatment. The major factor has been shown to be the hesitation from the onset of symptoms to the decision to seek medical assistance.

Once the decision to seek medical assistance has been made, the use of EMS has been shown to reduce the time to neurologic evaluation and subsequent treatment. Thus, EMS plays an important role in rapidly evaluating and transporting acute stroke patients to stroke-capable facilities.

When responding to patients with possible acute stroke, EMS providers should attempt to reduce the on-scene time in order to decrease the window from symptom onset to definitive treatment. Studies examining times-to-treatment in both ST-elevation myocardial infarction and acute stroke patients have shown that EMS "on-scene" time is a significant portion of the total prehospital time.[62-4] For patients with traumatic injuries, the National Association of EMTs has endorsed a goal of 10-minute scene times with limited scene interventions. *While there is no standard target scene-time for suspected stroke patients, it seems reasonable to treat stroke in the same time-critical fashion that we accord to trauma. There is early evidence that incorporating a scene-time limit into EMS protocols decreases scene-time for stroke patients.*[65]

While on scene, EMS providers must perform multiple tasks. In addition to performing the initial assessment, prehospital stroke screen and obtaining baseline vital signs, EMS providers should determine the time of symptom onset as well as a detailed patient history. *The onset of symptom time is a key determinant in the management of the patient and EMS providers are in a unique position to ascertain this information from witnesses on scene. Providers should also obtain an accurate description of the patient's baseline behavior in order to determine the severity of acute deficits.*

Triage to stroke centers

In recent years, accrediting bodies have begun to determine which hospitals are best staffed and equipped to provide the most appropriate care for acute stroke patients.[66] Many studies have detailed the improvement in survival rates, quality of life and return to functional baseline when patients are cared for at dedicated stroke centers.[67-70] Not only must EMS professionals recognize stroke and deliver timely and appropriate care, they must become part of the stroke system of care by choosing appropriate destination facilities for their acute stroke patients. Rapid delivery of acute stroke patients to stroke centers capable of providing state-of-the-art stroke care results in improved recovery and return to functional capacity.[18, 71-3]
To achieve this goal, EMS systems should establish firm transport guidelines for providers as a part of stroke protocols which enable EMS providers to transport acute stroke patients to appropriate facilities. When such a facility is available within a reasonable transport interval, stroke patients who require hospitalization should be admitted there.

Prehospital notification of receiving hospital

The prehospital notification of the impending arrival of an acute stroke patient can significantly improve the delivery of timely stroke therapy such as thrombolytic medications.[18, 33, 74-8] McKinney *et al.* found that emergency department processing times improved by as much as 18 minutes when pre-notification occurred.[75] Patel found similar results in a retrospective study of a stroke registry.[79] Lin *et al.* studied prehospital notification in a national sample of stroke patients. They examined the effect of prehospital notification on emergency department processing times, such as how long it takes to get a CT scan or to activate the stroke team. They found that EMS hospital prenotification is associated with improved evaluation, timelier stroke treatment and more eligible patients treated with tissue plasminogen activator (TPA).[77] In a different study, Lin *et al.* found that prenotification varied widely from 0 percent in some hospitals to 100 percent in others. Variation by region was also notable, with Washington, DC facilities reporting 19.7 percent prenotification by EMS to 93.4 percent for Montana hospitals. Unfortunately, they also noted little change in EMS prenotification rates between 2003 and 2011 (58.0 to 67.3 percent).[76] Some investigators have begun to explore the feasibility of direct activation of stroke teams by EMS providers.[67, 71] This warrants further investigation.

Summary

Management of strokes is a medical emergency, and prehospital care plays a large role in getting eligible patients the reperfusion treatment they need. It begins with stroke recognition by 9-1-1 dispatch and by EMS providers, often assisted by the use of structured stoke assessment algorithms and stroke scales. And it extends through scene management including triage to a stroke center and prehospital notification. Several prehospital interventions are required to avoid worsening of the ischemic injury or complications of the ischemia, including hypoglycemia, hypoxia and blood pressure extremes. In all of these roles and more, prehospital care has a critical impact on outcomes of stroke patients.

Key issues for future investigation

1. The addition of stroke scales into the 9-1-1 telecommunicator's protocol for possible stroke is in its infancy and will require additional research to refine, validate and improve implementation of these 9-1-1 assessment tools.

2. There are many prehospital stroke scales in use, which is confusing for EMS medical directors and field providers. Only a few of these scales have been validated in actual field practice and most of them have poor test characteristics. Investigators will need to develop prehospital stroke scales with better sensitivity and specificity and then evaluate and validate these stroke scales in actual field practice.

3. Telemedicine is a developing assessment modality that may prove beneficial in the prehospital setting, but little research has been devoted to this topic to date.

4. The recommendations regarding prehospital blood pressure management are inferred from inpatient treatment. No quality studies exist to support a hypertensive level above which prehospital treatment should begin. Is there a level of hypertension that requires prehospital intervention?

5. While studies suggest routine use of oxygen without hypoxia in the treatment of stroke can have deleterious effects, no rigorous studies confirm these findings.

Is oxygen beneficial in severe stroke even without confirmed hypoxia?

6. Further research is required to find effective and safe neuroprotective agents. This could significantly decrease the time to first treatment in acute stroke if the agents are able to be administered in the prehospital setting.

7. The effects of hospital bypass in favor of stroke centers of care have been studied in the prehospital environment and appear promising. Additional work will be required to fully understand the long-term effects on patients, EMS systems and hospital systems of care.

8. In the case of ST-elevation myocardial infarction, EMS direct notification of cardiac teams has been demonstrated to improve time to delivery of life-saving treatment. EMS direct notification of stroke teams remains to be studied.

REFERENCES

1. National Institute of Neurological Disorders and Stroke (NINDS) (2013). NINDS stroke information page, available at www.ninds.nih.gov/disorders/stroke/stroke.htm.

2. Saver, J. L., Fonarow, G. C., Smith, E. E. *et al.* (2013). "Time to treatment with intravenous tissue plasminogen activator and outcome from acute ischemic stroke," *JAMA* 309(23): 2480–8.

3. Hoyert, D. L. and Xu, J. (2012). "Deaths: preliminary data for 2011," *National Vital Statistics Reports* 61(6): 1–52, available at www.cdc.gov/nchs/data/nvsr/nvsr61/nvsr61_06.pdf.

4. Go, A. S., Mozaffarian, D., Roger, V. L. *et al.* (2013). "Heart disease and stroke statistics – 2013 update: a report from the American Heart Association," *Circulation* 127(1): 143–52.

5. Heidenreich, P. A., Trogdon, J. G., Khavjou, O. A. *et al.* (2011). "Forecasting the future of cardiovascular disease in the United States: a policy statement from the American Heart Association," *Circulation* 123(8): 933–44.

6. Hankey, G. (1996). "Impact of treatment of people with transient ischaemic attack on stroke incidence and public health," *Cerebrovasc. Dis.* 6(Suppl. 1): 26–33.

7. Johnston, S. C., Gress, D. R., Browner, W. S. *et al.* (2000). "Short-term prognosis after emergency department diagnosis of TIA," *JAMA* 284(22): 2901–6.

8. Wu, C. M., McLaughlin, K., Lorenzetti, D. L. *et al.* (2007). "Early risk of stroke after transient ischemic attack: a systematic review and meta-analysis," *Arch. Intern. Med.* 167(22): 2417–22.

9. Giles, M. F. and Rothwell, P. M. (2007). "Risk of stroke early after transient ischaemic attack: a systematic review and meta-analysis," *Lancet Neurol.* 6(12): 1063–72.

10. Maio, R. F., Garrison, H. G., Spaite, D. W. *et al.* (1999). "Emergency medical services outcomes project I (EMSOP I): prioritizing conditions for outcomes research," *Ann. Emerg. Med.* 33(4): 423–32.

11. California Acute Stroke Pilot Registry (CASPR) Investigators (2005). "Prioritizing interventions to improve rates of thrombolysis for ischemic stroke," *Neurology* 64(4): 654–9.

12. Brice, J. H., Griswell, J. K., Delbridge, T. R. *et al.* (2002). "Stroke: from recognition by the public to management by emergency medical services," *Prehosp. Emerg. Care* 6(1): 99–107.

13. Rosamond, W. D., Evenson, K. R., Schroeder, E. B. *et al.* (2005). "Calling emergency medical services for acute stroke: a study of 9-1-1 tapes," *Prehosp. Emerg. Care* 9(1): 19–23.

14. Liferidge, A. T., Brice, J. H., Overby, B. A. *et al.* (2004). "The ability of laypersons to utilize the Cincinnati Prehospital Stroke Scale," *Prehosp. Emerg. Care* 8(4): 384–7.

15. Hurwitz, A. S., Brice, J. H., Overby, B. A. *et al.* (2005). "Directed use of the Cincinnati Prehospital Stroke Scale by laypersons," *Prehosp. Emerg. Care* 9(3): 292–6.

16. Ramanujam, P., Guluma, K. Z., Castillo, E. M. *et al.* (2008). "Accuracy of stroke recognition by emergency medical dispatchers and paramedics – San Diego experience," *Prehosp. Emerg. Care* 12(3): 307–13.

17. Krebes, S., Ebinger, M., Baumann, A. M. *et al.* (2012). "Development and validation of a dispatcher identification algorithm for stroke emergencies," *Stroke* 43(3): 776–81.

18. Quain, D. A., Parsons, M. W., Loudfoot, A. R. *et al.* (2008). "Improving access to acute stroke therapies: a controlled trial of organized pre-hospital and emergency care," *Med. J. Aust.* 189: 429–33.

19. National Institute of Neurological Disorders and Stroke (NINDS) (2013). "NIH stroke scale," available at www.ninds.nih.gov/doctors/NIH_Stroke_Scale_Booklet.pdf.

20. Brott, T., Adams, H. P., Olinger, C. P. *et al.* (1989). "Measurements of acute cerebral infarction: a clinical examination scale," *Stroke* 20(7): 864–70.

21. de Haan, R., Horn, J., Limburg, M. *et al.* (1993). "A comparison of five stroke scales with measures of disability, handicap, and quality of life," *Stroke* 24(8): 1178–81.

22. Kothari, R., Hall, K., Brott, T. *et al.* (1997). "Early stroke recognition: developing an out-of-hospital NIH stroke scale," *Acad. Emerg. Med.* 4(10): 986–90.

23. Kothari, R. U., Pancioli, A., Liu, T. *et al.* (1999). "Cincinnati Prehospital Stroke Scale: reproducibility and validity," *Ann. Emerg. Med.* 33(4): 373–8.

24. Frendl, D. M., Strauss, D. G., Underhill, B. K. *et al.* (2009). "Lack of impact of paramedic training and use of the Cincinnati prehospital stroke scale on stroke patient identification and on-scene time," *Stroke* 40(3): 754–6.

25. Kidwell, C. S., Saver, J. L., Schubert, G. B. *et al.* (1998). "Design and retrospective analysis of the Los Angeles Prehospital Stroke Screen (LAPSS)," *Prehosp. Emerg. Care* 2(4): 267–73.

26. Kidwell, C. S., Starkman, S. and Eckstein, M. (2000). "Identifying stroke in the field. Prospective validation of the Los Angeles Prehospital Stroke Screen (LAPSS)," *Stroke* 31(1): 71–6.

27. Ziegler, V., Rashid, A., Müller-Gorchs, M. *et al.* (2008). "Mobile computing systems in preclinical care of stroke," *Anaesthesist* 57(7): 677–85.

28. Studnek, J., Asimos, A., Dodds, J. *et al.* (2013). "Assessing the validity of the Cincinnati prehospital stroke scale and the medic prehospital assessment for code stroke in an urban emergency medical services agency," *Prehosp. Emerg. Care* 17(3): 348–53.

29. Hasegawa, Y., Sasaki, N., Yamada, K. *et al.* (2013). "Prediction of thrombolytic therapy after stroke-bypass transportation: the Maria prehospital stroke scale score," *J. Stroke Cerebrovasc. Dis.* 22(4): 514–19.

30. Nor, A. M., Davis, J., Sen, B. *et al.* (2005). "The Recognition of Stroke in the Emergency Room (ROSIER) scale: development and validation of a stroke recognition instrument," *Lancet Neurol.* 4(11): 727–34.

31. Mingfeng, H., Zhixin, W., Qihong, G. *et al.* (2012). "Validation of the use of the ROSIER scale in prehospital assessment of stroke," *Ann. Indian Acad. Neurol.* 15(3): 191–5.

32. Bray, J. E., Martin, J., Cooper, G. *et al.* (2005). "Paramedic identification of stroke: community validation of the Melbourne ambulance stroke screen," *Cerebrovasc. Dis.* 20(1): 28–33.

33. Bray, J. E., Coughlan, K., Barger, B. *et al.* (2010). "Paramedic diagnosis of stroke: examining long-term use of the Melbourne Ambulance Stroke Screen (MASS) in the field," *Stroke* 41(7): 1363–6.

34. Harbison, J., Hossain, O., Jenkinson, D. *et al.* (2003). "Diagnostic accuracy of stroke referrals from primary care, emergency room physicians, and ambulance staff using the face arm speech test," *Stroke* 34(1): 71–6.

35. Nor, A. M., McAllister, C., Louw, S. J. *et al.* (2004). "Agreement between ambulance paramedic- and physician-recorded neurological signs with Face Arm Speech Test (FAST) in acute stroke patients," *Stroke* 35(6): 1355–9.

36. Lacombe, D. M., Gordon, D. L., Issenberg, S. B. *et al.* (2000). "Stroke on the MEND," *J. Emerg. Med. Serv.* 25(10): 32–41.

37. Brotons, A. A., Motola, I., Rivera, H. F. *et al.* (2012). "Correlation of the Miami Emergency Neurologic Deficit (MEND) exam performed in the field by paramedics with an abnormal NIHSS and final diagnosis of stroke for patients airlifted from the scene," *Stroke* 43: A3468.

38. Chenkin, J., Gladstone, D. J., Verbeek, P. R. *et al.* (2009). "Predictive value of the Ontario prehospital stroke screening tool for the identification of patients with acute stroke," *Prehosp. Emerg. Care* 13(2): 153–9.

39. Hepburn, D. A., Deary, I. J., Frier, B. M. *et al.* (1991). "Symptoms of acute insulin-induced hypoglycemia in humans with and without IDDM. Factor-analysis approach," *Diabetes Care* 14(11): 949–57.

40. Wallis, W. E., Donaldson, I., Scott, R. S. *et al.* (1985). "Hypoglycemia masquerading as cerebrovascular disease (hypoglycemic hemiplegia)," *Ann. Neurol.* 18: 510–12.

41. Gatto, E. M., Fernandez Pardal, M. M. and Fueyo, G. (1992). "Hypoglycemic hemiparesis," *Neurologia* 7(2): 77–9.

42. Foster, J. W. and Hart, R. G. (1987). "Hypoglycemic hemiplegia: two cases and a clinical review," *Stroke* 18(5): 944–6.

43. Megarbane, B., Deye, N., Bloch, V. *et al.* (2007). "Intentional overdose with insulin: prognostic factors and toxicokinetic / toxicodynamic profiles," *Crit. Care* 11(5): R115.

44. Jauch, E. C., Cucchiara, B., Adeoye, O. *et al.* (2010). "Part 11: adult stroke: 2010 American Heart Association Guidelines for Cardiopulmonary Resuscitation and Emergency Cardiovascular Care," *Circulation* 122(Suppl. 3): S818–28.

45. Gilmore, R. M., Miller, S. J. and Stead, L. G. (2005). "Severe hypertension in the emergency department patient," *Emerg. Med. Clin. N. Am.* 23(4): 1141–58.

46. Wallace, J. D. and Levy, L. L. (1981). "Blood pressure after stroke," *JAMA* 246(19): 2177.

47. Jain, A. R., Bellolio, M. F. and Stead, L. G. (2009). "Treatment of hypertension in acute ischemic stroke," *Curr. Treatment Options Neurol.* 11(2): 120–5.

48. Leonardi-Bee, J., Bath, P. M. and Phillips, S. J. (2002). "Blood pressure and clinical outcomes in the International Stroke Trial," *Stroke* 33(5): 1315–20.

49. Jauch, E. C., Saver, J. L., Adams, H. P. *et al.* (2013). "Guidelines for the early management of patients with acute ischemic stroke: a guideline for healthcare professionals from the American Heart Association/ American Stroke Association," *Stroke* 44(3): 870–947.

50. Vemmos, K. N., Tsivgoulis, G., Spengos, K. *et al.* (2004). "U-shaped relationship between mortality and admission blood pressure in patients with acute stroke," *J. Int. Med.* 255(2): 257–65.

51. Stead, L. G., Gilmore, R. M., Decker, W. W. *et al.* (2005). "Initial emergency department blood pressure as predictor of survival after acute ischemic stroke," *Neurology* 65(8): 1179–83.

52. Willmot, M., Leonardi-Bee, J. and Bath, P. M. (2004). "High blood pressure in acute stroke and subsequent outcome: a systematic review," *Hypertension* 43(1): 18–24.

53. Oliveira-Filho, J., Silva, S. C. S. and Trabuco, C. C. (2003). "Detrimental effect of blood pressure reduction in the first 24 hours of acute stroke onset," *Neurology* 61(8): 1047–51.

54. Adams, H., Del Zoppo, G., Alberts, M. *et al.* (2007). "Guidelines for the early management of patients with acute ischemic stroke," *Circulation* 115: e478–e534.

55. Kue, R. and Steck, A. (2012). "Acute ischemic stroke prehospital diagnosis and management of patients with acute stroke," *Emerg. Med. Clin. NA* 30(3): 617–35.

56. Ronning, O. M. and Guldvog, B. (1999). "Should stroke victims routinely receive supplemental oxygen? A quasi-randomized controlled trial," *Stroke* 30(10): 2033–7.

57. Kety, S. S. and Schmidt, C. F. (1948). "The effects of altered tensions of carbon dioxide and oxygen on cerebral blood flow and cerebral oxygen consumption of normal young men," *J. Clin. Invest.* 27(4): 484–92.

58. Hallenbeck, J. and Dutka, A. (1990). "Background review and current concepts of reperfusion injury," *Arch. Neurol.* 47(11): 1245–54.

59. Branson, R. D. and Johannigman, J. A. (2013). "Pre-hospital oxygen therapy," *Respir. Care* 58(1): 86–94.

60. Xu, S. Y. and Pan, S. Y. (2013). "The failure of animal models of neuroprotection in acute ischemic stroke to translate to clinical efficacy," *Med. Sci. Monit. Basic Res.* 19: 37–45.

61. Horn, J., de Haan, R. J., Vermeulen, M. *et al.* (2001). "Very early Nimodipine use in stroke (VENUS): a randomized, double-blind, placebo-controlled trial," *Stroke* 32(2): 461–5.

62. Chughtai, H., Ratner, D., Pozo, M. *et al.* (2011). "Prehospital delay and its impact on time to treatment in ST-elevation myocardial infarction," *Am. J. Emerg. Med.* 29(4): 396–400.

63. Herlitz, J., Wireklintsundstrom, B., Bang, A. *et al.* (2010). "Early identification and delay to treatment in myocardial infarction and stroke: differences and similarities," *Scand. J. Trauma Resusc. Emerg. Med.* 18: 48.

64. Keskin, O., Kalemoglu, M. and Ulusoy, R. (2005). "A clinic investigation into prehospital and emergency department delays in acute stroke care," *Med. Princ. Prac.* 14(6): 408–12.

65. Patel, M. D., Brice, J. H., Moss, C. *et al.* (2013). "Association of emergency medical services stroke protocols with minimizing on-scene time for stroke patients," *Circ. Cardiovasc. Qual. Outcomes* 6: A210.

66. Song, S. and Saver, J. (2012). "Growth of regional acute stroke systems of care in the United States in the first decade of the 21st century," *Stroke* 43(7): 1975–8.

67. Douglas, V. C., Tong, D. C., Gillum, L. A. *et al.* (2005). "Do the Brain Attack Coalition's criteria for stroke centers improve care for ischemic stroke?" *Neurology* 64(3): 422–7.

68. Chapman, K. M., Woolfenden, A. R., Graeb, D. *et al.* (2000). "Intravenous tissue plasminogen activator for acute ischemic stroke: a Canadian hospital's experience," *Stroke* 31(12): 2920–4.

69. Merino, J. G., Silver, B., Wong, E. *et al.* (2002). "Extending tissue plasminogen activator use to community and rural stroke patients," *Stroke* 33(1): 141–6.

70. Riopelle, R. J., Howse, D. C., Bolton, C. *et al.* (2001). "Regional access to acute ischemic stroke intervention," *Stroke* 32(3): 652–5.

71. Gladstone, D. J., Rodan, L. H., Sahlas, D. J. *et al.* (2009). "A citywide prehospital protocol increases access to stroke thrombolysis in Toronto," *Stroke* 40(12): 3841–4.

72. Garnett, A. R., Marsden, D. L., Parsons, M. W. *et al.* (2010). "The rural Prehospital Acute Stroke Triage (PAST) trial protocol: a controlled trial for rapid facilitated transport of rural acute stroke patients to a regional stroke centre," *Int. J. Stroke* 5(6): 506–13.

73. Gropen, T., Magdon-Ismail, Z., Day, D. *et al.* (2009). "Regional implementation of the stroke systems of care model: recommendations of the northeast cerebrovascular consortium," *Stroke* 40(5): 1793–802.

74. Kim, S. K., Lee, S. Y., Bae, H. J. *et al.* (2009). "Pre-hospital notification reduced the door-to-needle time for IV t-PA in acute ischaemic stroke," *Eur. J. Neurol.* 16(12): 1331–5.

75. McKinney, J. S., Mylavarapu, K., Lane, J. *et al.* (2013). "Hospital prenotification of stroke patients by emergency medical services improves stroke time targets," *J. Stroke Cerebrovasc. Dis.* 22(2): 113–18.

76. Lin, C. B., Peterson, E. D., Smith, E. E. *et al.* (2012a). "Patterns, predictors, variations, and temporal trends in emergency medical service hospital prenotification for acute ischemic stroke," *J. Am. Heart Assoc.* 1, e-pub: e002345.

77. Lin, C. B., Peterson, E. D., Smith, E. E. *et al.* (2012b). "Emergency medical service hospital prenotification is associated with improved evaluation and treatment of acute ischemic stroke," *Circ. Cardiovasc. Qual. Outcomes* 5(4): 514–22.

78. Abdullah, A. R., Smith, E. E., Biddinger, P. D. *et al.* (2008). "Advance hospital notification by EMS in acute stroke is associated with shorter door-to-computed tomography time and increased likelihood of administration of tissue-plasminogen activator," *Prehosp. Emerg. Care* 12(4): 426–31.

79. Patel, M. D., Rose, K. M., O'Brien, E. C. *et al.* (2011). "Prehospital notification by emergency medical services reduces delays in stroke evaluation: findings from the North Carolina stroke care collaborative," *Stroke* 42(8): 2263–8.

Chapter 5

Spinal cord injury

J. Stephen Huff and Eric Jaeger

Recommendations

High quality

There are insufficient data to support high quality recommendations for this topic.

Moderate quality

1. EMS systems should implement spine assessment protocols such as the NEXUS criteria or Canadian C-spine rule to identify patients at extremely low risk of cervical spine injuries and safely forego cervical spine immobilization.

2. The provider may safely forego cervical immobilization in patients that exhibit no altered mental status (i.e. patient is alert), no evidence of intoxication, no painful injury that would distract the patient from a cervical spine injury (i.e. an injury that would prevent the patient from reliably participating in the assessment), have no midline cervical

Prehospital Care of Neurologic Emergencies, ed. Todd J. Crocco and Michael R. Sayre. Published by Cambridge University Press. © Cambridge University Press 2014.

pain or tenderness on palpation, and no focal neurological deficit, i.e. numbness, tingling or weakness in any extremity.
3. Use caution when applying assessment protocols in patients older than 65 years of age.
4. Do NOT use steroids to treat patients with acute spinal cord injury.

Low quality

1. To limit spinal movement, EMS providers should immobilize patients at risk for spinal injury, i.e. those patients not meeting criteria for a validated spine assessment clearance guideline.
2. Oral intubation with RSI techniques and cervical stabilization should be used when needed for respiratory support.
3. Consider preferentially transporting patients with suspected clinically significant spinal cord injuries to Level I or II trauma centers. For patients with multi-system trauma, including pelvic trauma or suspected internal hemorrhage with hypotension, consider transport directly to a Level I trauma center.
4. There is insufficient evidence to make a specific recommendation for performing a particular technique or using a specific device for performing spinal immobilization.

Overview

The consequences of a spinal cord injury can be catastrophic. Motor vehicle accidents, falls and other mechanisms of injury with the potential to cause spinal cord injuries are common. Over 1 million patients with a suspected spine injury are transported annually by emergency medical services in the United States and Canada.[1, 2] Fortunately, only a very small percentage (0.5 to 3 percent) of these patients are ultimately found to have a spinal fracture, and an even smaller percentage are clinically significant (0.05 to 1 percent).[1–5] For patients who have sustained spinal trauma, management has focused on preventing secondary injury by immobilizing the spine and supporting adequate perfusion and oxygenation. Faced with reconciling the low incidence of injury with the potentially devastating consequences of a cord injury, providers have historically treated all patients as if they had an actual injury based solely on the mechanism of injury even in the absence of clinical signs or symptoms. This has resulted in a *significant over-triage of suspected spine injury.*[1] Additionally, although the EMS interventions for spine injuries are in wide use, they have not been rigorously studied. Use of these interventions, especially in a patient without a spine injury, is time-consuming, expensive and may be harmful.

The spine consists of the spinal cord and the vertebral column. The vertebral column is composed of the vertebrae, the intervertebral discs and associated ligamentous structures, and provides protection and support for the spinal cord. The spine is divided into the cervical spine, consisting of seven vertebrae (C1 to C7), the thoracic spine, consisting of twelve vertebrae (T1 to T12), the lumbar spine, consisting of five vertebrae (L1 to L5), the sacrum, consisting of five fused vertebrae, and the coccyx, consisting of four fused vertebrae.

The spinal cord is part of the central nervous system and extends from the brainstem to the upper lumbar vertebra. The spinal cord courses within the spinal canal bound by the posterior elements of the vertebrae, ligamentous structures, the bodies of the vertebrae and the intervertebral discs.

Primary injuries are direct injuries that occur at the time of the traumatic event and include fractures of the spinal column and direct injuries to the spinal cord. The pathophysiology of injury is more complicated than the simple mechanics of bone fragments impacting the spinal cord. Additional mechanisms of primary injury include impingement on the cord by soft tissue elements such as discs and ligaments, and vascular injury of vessels supplying the spinal cord.

Secondary injuries arise in the minutes to hours following the initial trauma. The movement of unstable fractures may cause injury to the cord, and preventing such injuries is the focus of current EMS practice. Important mechanisms of secondary injury include hypoxia and hypoperfusion, which often contribute to neurologic impairment. Additionally, a complex biochemical cascade often occurs following an injury that results in inflammation, hemorrhage and edema, worsening neuronal injury.

Spinal fractures are identified by the anatomic region of the fracture: cervical, thoracic or lumbar. Fractures of the spine may occur at any vertebral level, but *the cervical spine is especially vulnerable to injury* because of the smaller size of the cervical vertebrae and supporting ligaments, and movement of the cervical spine influenced by the relatively heavy head. Spinal fractures are additionally categorized as mechanically stable or unstable. The currently prevailing view is that unstable fractures present a greater risk of secondary injury, as moving bone fragments may injure the cord. This view underlies the practice of spinal immobilization, which seeks to minimize movement of the spine during EMS management.[2] A competing view holds that most cord injuries, even in the context of unstable fractures, occur during the initial accident.[2, 5]

Spinal cord injuries are feared because of the devastating loss of function and limited recovery with many such injuries. *Spinal cord injury patterns are either complete or partial* (see Table 5.1). Complete or transverse injuries are the most common pattern and result in loss of all motor and sensory function below the level of injury. Incomplete cord injury patterns also occur. Central cord syndrome affects the upper extremities out of proportion to the lower extremities. Although patients with spinal cord injuries typically exhibit a loss of function, those with central cord injuries may complain of burning hands in the upper extremities. Patients with unusual hemisection or half-cord injury patterns may show loss of motor function (i.e. paralysis) on the same side of the body as the injury, and loss of pain and temperature sensations on the other side of the body. In general, incomplete spinal cord injuries have a better prognosis than complete spinal cord injuries.[6]

Hypotension from neurogenic shock may follow cervical spinal cord injuries when loss of vascular tone causes a form of distributive shock. *Hypotension from spinal cord injury is a diagnosis of exclusion* and the provider should suspect that other injuries are more likely causing the hypotension.

Table 5.1 Syndromes

Syndrome	Sensory	Motor	Sphincter impairment
Transverse cord syndrome – complete	Loss of sensation below level of injury	Loss of motor function below level of cord injury	Sphincter control lost. Priapism may be present
Central cord syndrome	Variable loss	Upper extremity weakness greater than lower extremity weakness	Variable
Brown-Sequard or hemisection syndrome	Loss of position sense and vibration sense on same side of injury. Loss of pain and temperature sense on opposite side of injury	Motor function loss on same side as cord injury	Variable
Anterior cord syndrome	Vibration and positions sense preserved. Loss of pain and touch sensation below level of injury	Motor loss or weakness below level of cord injury	Variable
Conus medullaris and cauda equina syndromes	Complete or patchy sensory loss may be present (saddle anesthesia)	Weakness in legs	Sphincter control impaired

Key challenges

The first challenge to the EMS provider is recognition and assessment of potential spine injuries. Once a spine injury is suspected, traditional management involves preventing secondary injury with spine immobilization to limit movement and mitigate further injury. A fundamental question for providers is: Should all patients be immobilized, or is it possible to selectively identify and immobilize patients that are at risk from a clinically significant spine injury? Additionally, the role of neuroprotective agents – specifically steroids – has been studied extensively.

Examination of patients with possible spine injuries

Examination of the patient with suspected spine or spinal cord injury by the EMS provider involves an assessment of motor and sensory function. Signs and symptoms of a potential spine injury include:

- pain or tenderness along the spine whether with movement, palpation or if spontaneously present;
- pain or tenderness to palpation in the center of the patient's back;
- paresthesia or anesthesia (i.e. tingling, numbness or loss of sensation);
- paralysis or weakness (unilateral or bilateral);
- soft tissue injury that may involve injury to the spine;
- loss of bowel or bladder control, priapism.

For potentially serious injuries, the time-limited nature of the interaction is such that assessment will be brief. However, much of the needed assessment may be accomplished by observing responses to clear commands for movement of the lower extremities, the upper extremities and a rough grading of motor function as normal, weak or absent. Sensory assessment may be limited to a query regarding perception of tactile stimulation. Formal sensory testing and assessment of reflexes, although potentially informative, is beyond the scope of most EMS field examinations. *With cervical injuries, motor function may be so impaired that respirations become inadequate and respiratory support becomes necessary.*

It is vitally important that the EMS provider perform a brief examination to assess disability in the injured patient. In the patient with altered mental status from injury or intoxicants, accurate assessment simply may not be possible. Erroneous notation that the patient was moving all extremities after an injury puts all providers at potential medicolegal risk when the case is retrospectively reviewed.

Which patients do not require immobilization despite the presence of a mechanism of injury that could potentially cause spine injury?

It has long been axiomatic that the spine should be immobilized whenever a patient experiences trauma that has the potential to cause spine injury. This has been the standard of EMS care for decades. The decision to immobilize was based solely on the mechanism of injury (i.e. the kinematics of the trauma) without regard to the actual risk of injury or the patient's clinical condition. However, there are emerging questions about proper selection of patients for immobilization, and even the value of prehospital immobilization.[1, 2, 4, 5, 7]

For many years, the standard of care for all of these patients was "full spinal immobilization," which involves applying a rigid cervical collar and fully immobilizing the patient to a hard backboard.[1, 2, 4, 5, 7] Given the potentially catastrophic consequences of a spine injury, the EMS approach to immobilization has remained conservative, requiring immobilization even in the absence of any clinical signs or symptoms of injury.[2, 4] This practice has not been validated by high quality evidence demonstrating that it protects patients from further injury.[1–5, 7–9] One small study, a retrospective chart review that compared patients at the University of Mexico who received immobilization with patients at the University of Malaya who did not, concluded that patients who were immobilized had worse outcomes even after correcting for mechanism of injury.[8]

It has also been recognized that *spinal immobilization has significant potential disadvantages*, including harm caused directly by immobilization, delays in treatment or transport, and increased exposure to radiation from unnecessary radiographic studies.[1–5, 8–10] The process of immobilization may increase manipulation of the cervical spine (when compared with no immobilization), and cause respiratory compromise, pressure-related tissue breakdown, increased intracranial pressure and even additional spinal cord injury.[1-4] Unnecessary spinal immobilization consumes important on-scene time that may delay transport or be better used for other procedures.[1, 10] Additionally, over-immobilization contributes to emergency department crowding and may result in patients being exposed to excess radiation and expense as a consequence of unnecessary radiographic studies.[1]

Because of the possible detrimental effects of unnecessary immobilization and the lack of definitive evidence of its utility, multiple researchers have examined whether EMS providers could utilize a clinical spinal assessment protocol to selectively immobilize patients at risk for significant injury, rather than immobilize all patients based only on mechanism of injury.[1, 2, 4, 11, 12] The goal of these studies was to determine whether the rate of over-immobilization could be safely reduced. These studies have demonstrated that *EMS providers are capable of determining whether a trauma patient has a low risk of spinal cord injury and thus does not require immobilization.*[1, 2, 4] Under these protocols, patients who have experienced a mechanism that might injure the spine are fully immobilized unless they meet several specific criteria that allow exclusion from immobilization. Even where a patient meets the criteria for avoiding immobilization, many of these protocols permit the provider to immobilize the patient if it is warranted in their clinical judgment.

Most of the current EMS field protocols are derived from the NEXUS study published in 2000,[13] as well as the Canadian C-spine rule (CCR) study published 2001.[14] These groundbreaking studies examined whether emergency physicians could identify patients at low risk for a clinically significant injury in order to avoid unnecessary radiographic examination.[13-15] *The NEXUS and CCR studies did not address selective spinal immobilization by EMS providers in the prehospital environment.* The goal of both studies was to describe a simple set of clinical criteria for spinal injury that could be rapidly performed by a physician and identify patients without the need for imaging or further tests. One principal distinction between the NEXUS and CCR protocols is that the NEXUS criteria can be applied regardless of severity of mechanism of injury, whereas the CCR excludes patients who have suffered a "dangerous mechanism of injury" (defined below).[14, 15] A second key distinction is that the NEXUS protocol is applied to patients of all ages, whereas the Canadian C-spine study excludes patients over 65 years of age. These studies demonstrated that emergency physicians could successfully determine which patients did not require imaging to exclude fractures.

Recognizing the potential utility of these assessment protocols to reduce the over-immobilization of trauma patients in the prehospital environment, many systems in the United States adopted EMS field protocols for selectively immobilizing patients who had potentially suffered a spine injury. Although not validated in the prehospital environment, medical directors reasoned that EMS providers would be able to apply the criteria in the field to identify patients at low risk for a clinically significant cervical spine injury. Subsequent studies have validated the application of these protocols by EMS providers. While the clinical criteria vary among studies, the NEXUS exclusion criteria have been widely studied and are incorporated in many EMS assessment protocols in the United States. Under these protocols, EMS providers may elect not to immobilize patients who meet all of the following exclusion criteria. The main purpose of the first three criteria is to ensure that a reliable examination can be performed.[4] The latter two criteria are indicators of potentially significant spine injury.

- no altered mental status (i.e. patient is alert);[1, 2, 4, 7, 12–15]
- no intoxication;[2, 4, 7, 12, 13]
- no painful injury that would distract the patient from a cervical spine injury;[2, 7, 13]
- no midline cervical pain or tenderness on palpation;[1, 2, 4, 7, 12–15]
- no focal neurological deficit, i.e. numbness, tingling or weakness in any extremity.[1, 2, 4, 7, 12–15]

Prehospital studies have concluded that the benefits of reducing over-immobilization outweigh the risks that a patient with a clinically important injury will be missed.[1, 2, 4, 12] While some studies have reported sensitivities as high as 99 to 100 percent in identifying unstable fractures,[1, 12, 13] others have reported lower sensitivity (but have nonetheless urged implementation).[4, 11] Seeking to achieve more consistent outcomes, as well as devise a tool that is readily applied by EMS providers and yields repeatable results in the field, researchers have studied revised versions of the original NEXUS and CCR criteria.

While the original NEXUS study reported sensitivities of 99.6 percent, the authors of the Canadian C-spine study reported that their examination of the NEXUS criteria yielded a much lower sensitivity of 90.7 percent.[13, 15] There is reason to believe, however, that this may not have reflected an accurate application of the NEXUS criteria.[16–18]

Presence of a painful, distracting injury

The requirement that the patient have no painful, distracting injury in order to avoid immobilization has proven to be challenging to apply, in part because it is not well defined. Lack of a clear definition makes it difficult to study with rigor and it has caused confusion among EMS providers.[14–16] The authors of the NEXUS study specifically chose not to define "distracting" injury, preferring instead to leave this to the clinical judgment of the providers performing the assessment.[13] It seems clear that this criterion is intended to include only injuries that produce significant pain that would prevent the patient from reliably participating in the remainder of the assessment. Some studies have addressed this ambiguity by defining narrower categories of more specific injuries as exclusion criteria.[4, 12] For example, Stroh *et al.* only immobilize patients who have suffered significant multi-system trauma or severe head or facial trauma; both of these injuries would presumably qualify as painful, distracting injuries.[12] Domeier *et al.* only immobilize patients who have a suspected extremity fracture proximal to the wrist or ankle.[4]

High risk mechanism of injury

A key question in utilizing spinal assessment protocols has been whether they may be applied to patients who have experienced a high risk mechanism of injury. For example, if a patient is involved in a rollover motor vehicle crash (MVC) and is unrestrained but meets all of the criteria, might the patient be transported without spinal immobilization, or is the nature of the mechanism sufficiently high risk that the patient should be immobilized, regardless of the apparent lack of injury? *Study protocols based on the NEXUS criteria can be applied, and immobilization avoided, regardless of the severity of the mechanism of injury.*[2, 4, 12, 13] The Canadian C-spine rule, in contrast, requires immobilization for all patients who have suffered a "dangerous mechanism of injury." "Dangerous mechanism of injury" is arbitrarily defined in the study as a fall from greater than 1 meter (5 stairs), diving or other axial load to the head, high speed MVC (>100 km/hr), ejection or rollover, or injury associated with a motorized recreational vehicle or bicycle collision.[1, 14, 15]

In the Canadian C-spine rule study, patients were considered to be at low risk for injury if they were alert (GCS = 15) and stable, and: (i) were younger than 65, had no paresthesias, had not suffered a dangerous mechanism of injury; and (ii) were able to have their cervical range of motion safely assessed due to the presence of one or more factors suggesting low risk; and (iii) could rotate their neck 45 degrees left and right. Low risk factors were: simple rear-end MVC, ambulatory on-scene, no neck pain, no pain during midline palpation.

In 2003, Steill *et al.* compared the Canadian C-spine rule with the NEXUS criteria.[15] Steill was also the lead investigator on the original 2001 Canadian C-spine rule. Vaillancourt examined the Canadian rule in the prehospital environment,[1] and in 2011 proposed additional prehospital studies of the rule.[19]

Age

The majority of assessment protocols do not use age as part of assessment criteria. The Canadian C-spine rule study excluded enrollment of patients aged greater than 65.[1, 14, 15] Studies have found increased occult spine injury in elderly patients, and a higher failure rate of study protocols.[2, 11, 12] Burton *et al.* note that excluding patients over 60 would have yielded a sensitivity of 100 percent for unstable fractures. It remains unclear, however, whether routinely immobilizing these patients yields improved clinical outcomes, especially as the harm associated with immobilization is likely greater in older patients.[2] A few study protocols excluded patients younger than 16; this appeared to be a limitation of the study design, rather than a conclusion that protocols would not be effective with pediatric patients.[4, 14] The NEXUS criteria have been evaluated in children and found to be reliable when applied by emergency physicians.[18, 20] Some EMS protocols in the United States have applied the NEXUS criteria only to children older than a certain age. Recent guidelines for spinal imaging in pediatric patients apply the criteria to children aged 9 and older.[18] More research is needed to refine and confirm the effectiveness of assessment protocols to pediatric patients.

Head rotation

The Canadian C-spine rule also requires that the patient be able to rotate the head left and right without provoking midline cervical pain or tenderness.[1, 14, 15] Many EMS field protocols that have implemented NEXUS-like criteria have included head rotation as an additional factor. While it has not been expressly validated as part of a published study in combination with the other NEXUS criteria, given that the intention of the assessment protocols is to be conservative in excluding immobilization, the addition of this criterion seems appropriate.

Proper application of assessment protocol

Stroh *et al.* required immobilization for patients who suffered loss of consciousness caused by trauma.[12]

In studies where patients with spinal fractures were not immobilized, some patients with injuries were not identified because EMS providers improperly applied the assessment protocol. Myers *et al.* noted that 9 of 42 patients (20 percent) who had spinal fractures should have been immobilized under the study protocol, but were not. He recommended continuous training and the implementation of quality assurance mechanisms.[11] It remains possible, however, that a different protocol might have yielded fewer missed fractures; that is, that the failure may have been a result of protocol design rather than one of training or performance.

For patients deemed to need spinal immobilization, what is the best method?

The goal of immobilization is to move the patient into a fully neutral, in-line position.[21] This position is believed to minimize the risk of secondary injury, although there is little firm evidence, since the concept is not well defined.[21, 22]

The patient is in the neutral, in-line position when he or she is facing straight-ahead and the patient's ears, shoulders and pelvis are in the same plane, with the patient's nose, chest, abdomen and feet facing forward and his or her arms at his or her side. Although high-level evidence for benefit does not exist, the process is described in this section for completeness.

Immobilization involves a series of steps that begin with manual stabilization during the initial assessment and extend through to full immobilization on a long spine board, ultimately concluding with the transfer of care at the emergency department. The determination of whether or not the patient requires full immobilization is made during this process. The equipment used to perform immobilization includes a rigid cervical collar, a long spine board with straps and blocks on either side of the head.[7, 21, 22] Patients who have just experienced significant trauma may be very anxious and uncomfortable. In addition to focusing on treatment priorities, efforts should be made to reassure and maintain frequent communication with the patient, since spinal immobilization procedures often cause further pain and discomfort.

If immobilization is deemed to be necessary, the following sequence of actions follows standard recommendations. Immediately upon approaching the patient, the head should be stabilized manually to limit further spine motion during assessment and immobilization. For patients who are conscious and alert and moving their heads without distress, direct the patient to look straight ahead and avoid turning the head. Explain that you will be placing your hands gently on either side of their head to protect their spine. Patients often have a very difficult time keeping their heads motionless, as they reflexively shake their heads yes and no and turn toward sounds or people they want to address. No traction should be applied during manual stabilization. The provider providing immobilization is often positioned behind the patient, but immobilization can also be accomplished while standing in front of the patient, which may facilitate communication.

Patients who are unconscious should be routinely immobilized, as should all patients who do not meet all of the exclusion criteria contained in the assessment protocol.[1, 2, 4, 7] For unconscious patients, initially maintain head position as found. Then gently move the head into the neutral in-line position stopping if meeting resistance or the patient exhibits discomfort. Once manual stabilization has been established, it should be maintained until the patient has been fully immobilized to a long spine board or similar device.

For conscious and alert patients, once manual stabilization has been achieved, providers may use a spinal assessment protocol to determine whether the patient requires full immobilization. Conscious patients at this stage often seek to refuse immobilization, either because they believe themselves to be uninjured or because they are anxious about the confined nature of immobilization. It is important to explain to the patient the benefits of the proposed treatment (protecting their spine from injury) and the risks of refusing treatment (possible catastrophic spinal cord injury).

Should the patient experience increased pain or the provider encounters resistance during the process of moving the patient into the neutral position, stop and reassess. Pain or resistance could indicate that movement is exacerbating the injury, and consideration should be given to immobilizing the patient in the position found. For example, if a patient is found on his side in a curled position, and experiences pain when an attempt is made to place him in a neutral position, the patient should be immobilized in a position of comfort that as nearly as possible approximates the neutral, in-line position. This may require improvisation by the provider. Lastly, patients with a grossly deformed spine should be immobilized as found.

After manual stabilization has been established and the cervical spine assessed, a rigid cervical collar should be applied. The cervical collar is thought to reduce the risk of further injury by limiting cervical motion and reducing axial loading. As with other immobilization techniques, very little research has examined the utility of cervical collars or any manufacturer's specific collar.[7, 21, 23, 24] Cervical collars are not benign interventions. Patients often find the collars very uncomfortable, which may increase their anxiety. Cervical collars apply an axial distractive force which may be inappropriate for injuries that are unstable with distraction.[25] Collars may increase intracranial pressure and decrease cerebral perfusion.[21, 26, 27] There is insufficient evidence to recommend a specific type of cervical collar.[21, 23] Given the variety of collars available, providers should follow the manufacturer's instructions for applying the collar. It is important to select the appropriate size collar since an improperly sized collar will be ineffective and may cause increased discomfort and further harm. For some patients, it will be impossible to locate an appropriately sized collar. For example, with obese patients, even the so-called "no neck" collar may not fit appropriately. In this event, a blanket roll secured on either side of the head may be effective. In the absence of a cervical collar, extra care must be taken to immobilize the patient onto the long spine board in a manner that will minimize cervical spine movement. Manual stabilization should be maintained even after a cervical collar has been applied; the collar is an adjunct that does not ensure immobilization.

The next step in the process is securing the patient to a long spine board or other immobilization device.[7, 21, 23] While other devices have been proposed, the rigid long spine board remains the de facto standard.[7, 21] The rigid board is uncomfortable for patients.[7, 23] It may also not result in in-line stabilization unless padding is added at the head.[21] Without introducing undue delay, carefully plan and coordinate moving the patient to minimize additional manipulation of the patient's spine during the process.[7] If the patient is found supine on the ground, the process may be straightforward. It has been traditional to use the log roll technique, but no large, published studies have validated this.[7, 21] Alternative techniques that have been suggested or studied include the lift-and-slide.[21, 24, 28] Properly performing these techniques requires multiple providers.[7, 21] For patients in small spaces such as a small bathroom or motor vehicle, the process is often more complex and avoiding manipulation of the spine is difficult. It has been suggested that patients who

self-extricate undergo less spinal movement than patients
extricated onto a long spine board. To insure coordination
among providers, the person providing manual stabilization
usually directs the process.[7] If the log roll technique is used,
the patient's back should be assessed for injuries when the
patient is rolled up onto her side.

Once on the long spine board, the patient's body is secured
to the board, typically with straps.[7, 21] Before the straps are
applied, consideration should be given to removal of clothing
that may interfere with care or be difficult to remove once the
patient is fully immobilized to the board. Care should be taken
to ensure that side-to-side motion is minimized. When
securing older patients to a backboard, it is appropriate to pad
under the head and knees to provide comfort.[7] Straps must be
sufficiently tight to minimize movement, especially in
circumstances where the immobilized patient will need to
be carried any distance or tilted during the process. The
straps must not be so tight that they restrict the patient's
respirations.[21] The patient's arms are usually not secured with
the patient's body to the spine board; thus, it is important,
especially in the unconscious patient, to safeguard the
patient's arms and hands from injury. This can be
accomplished by gently securing the patient's hands together
on top of their chest or abdomen. After the straps are secured,
soft blocks are placed on either side of the patient's head
and one or more straps are used to secure the patient's head
and the blocks to the board.[7, 21] Before this is done, it is
common for the cervical collar to need readjustment. In some
EMS protocols, a brief neurological exam is repeated after

the patient has been secured. When this process is complete, manual stabilization may be released.

For patients who are in a motor vehicle, there is debate regarding the best process for moving the patient onto a long spine board.[29] To obtain optimal access to the patient for purposes of full immobilization, it is commonplace for rescue personnel to use power extrication tools (for example, the jaws of life) to disassemble and remove significant portions of the vehicle, including the doors, roof, dashboard or seats. Unfortunately, these techniques can introduce considerable delay in the care and transport of the patient. For patients who are in fact entrapped with a portion of their body physically restrained by the vehicle, this form of extrication is clearly necessary. When these techniques are employed primarily to facilitate immobilization, there is debate concerning any utility given that little evidence exists for the value of spinal immobilization itself.[5] This is particularly true for patients who are unconscious or may be unstable. For example, it may offer little benefit to a patient to protect the cervical spine if they become hypotensive or develop increased intracranial pressure during the delay.[5] For patients who can be rapidly extricated, albeit with increased motion of the spine, providers should carefully consider whether the benefits associated with obtaining better access to accomplish full immobilization outweigh the risks.[21] Definitive care for multi-system trauma patients is in the hospital, and the delay associated with extended on-scene operations may exacerbate patient morbidity and mortality.

After patients are transferred to the ambulance, providers must determine the most appropriate destination hospital. Providers should consider preferentially transporting patients with suspected clinically significant spinal cord injuries to Level I or II trauma centers.[7, 30] For patients with multi-system trauma, including pelvic trauma and suspected internal hemorrhage with hypotension, consider transport directly to a Level I trauma center.[7] Macias *et al.* found that transfer to a trauma care center is associated with reduced paralysis, possibly due to a higher surgical volume.[30]

Occasionally, patients who initially are determined to be at low risk of having a clinically significant injury develop midline neck pain during transport to the hospital or after they have been secured to the stretcher. EMS providers are then left with the conundrum of whether to stop the ambulance en route and immobilze the patient. Backboarding a patient who is already secured to the stretcher may expose the patient to more spinal manipulation than simply placing a collar on the patient and continuing to the hospital with the patient secured to the stretcher.

For pediatric patients with a potential spine injury, there are several additional considerations, including the capacity of very young patients to participate reliably in an assessment and the appropriate selection of immobilization equipment. As in so many areas of emergency medical research, there are few useful studies regarding pediatric patients with spinal trauma. In part, this arises from the fact that spinal injury in children, and especially clinically significant spinal injury, is exceedingly rare.

Pediatric patients constituted 3,065 (9 percent) of all NEXUS study patients.[20] Less than 1 percent (30 patients) had cervical spine injuries.[20] Only 4 of the 30 children with CSI were younger than 9 years and none was younger than 2 years.[20] The NEXUS decision instrument correctly identified all pediatric CSI victims in this study.[20] Unfortunately, because the injuries were so rare, the confidence interval was very large. Many EMS protocols elect to immobilize all children under age 9. As a consequence, the rate of over-triage is even higher in children than in adults. For children, spinal immobilization can be terrifying. In very young children (less than 2 years old), the patient may vigorously resist immobilization, perversely resulting in significant spinal movement as a consequence of the theoretically beneficial (but unproven) immobilization. Pediatric spinal trauma presents a research paradox. Because the injuries are so rare in children, it is exceedingly difficult to do a clinical trial with adequate power to resolve the important questions regarding immobilization in children definitively.

The primary rationale provided for not applying exclusion criteria to young children appears to be the concern that they may not be able to participate reliably in the spinal assessment. The literature does not contain high-level evidence for a specific age below which the use of exclusion criteria is unsupported.

Once the decision has been made to immobilize a child, the appropriate equipment must be utilized. Adult immobilization equipment is inappropriate for children. Cervical collars are available in various adjustable and non-adjustable pediatric sizes. There is no "one-size-fits-all" pediatric backboard for use with children. Adult backboards may be effective for older (for example, 13 years plus) or heavier children, but may not be used for younger children. Adult backboards typically have fixed position attachment points, making them too wide to immobilize children. Younger children have a proportionately larger occiput, often resulting in inappropriate cervical flexion on a flat surface. This latter issue can be addressed with padding under the patient's shoulders, but is better addressed with a correctly sized pediatric backboard that has a depression to correctly position the head. A persistent question has been whether child car seats can be used for spinal immobilization. Child car seats are not designed to maintain a child in the neutral in-line position. For younger children, car seats present the same issue with flexion that an adult backboard does. Older children seated upright will often slump forward. Finally, if the child's own car seat is to be used, it must first be confirmed that the car seat was not damaged in the accident that precipitated the need for EMS. In many cases today, ambulances carry child car seats since they are thought to be the only safe way to transport a child, but even ambulance car seats have the same disadvantages ascribed to other car seats. The question has persisted whether removing a child from an undamaged car seat results in more spinal movement than simply maintaining the patient in their own car seat. If the patient has already been removed from her car seat and immobilization is indicated, immobilize the child using a pediatric backboard or other device specifically designed for pediatric patients. If the patient has not been removed from the car seat and the car seat is undamaged and can be adequately secured to the stretcher (two independent belt paths are required to secure a car seat to the stretcher), then it may be appropriate to immobilize the patient in her car seat on the ambulance stretcher.

What resuscitation techniques are the best in the spinal-cord-injured patient?

A patient may suffer spinal cord injury in isolation or with additional traumatic injuries. Basic tenets of trauma resuscitation have been recently challenged and ideal management is controversial. Permissive hypotension is advocated by some for patients with multi-system trauma. The benefit of endotracheal intubation in the trauma patient has recently been challenged as well. Although these discussions are outside the scope of this chapter, these controversies impact recommendations for the treatment of spinal-cord-injured patients.

One axiom in spinal cord injury management is that multi-system trauma is assumed to be present until proven otherwise. With alteration in sensory and motor functions in most cord-injured patients, physical examination may be unreliable and vital signs may be difficult to interpret.

Assessment of the airway and appropriate intervention is a fundamental principle of trauma management. To open the airway, the jaw thrust maneuver is preferred, but head tilt, chin lift technique may be required if unable to open with jaw thrust.[31] Head tilt ideally is minimized. Simple maneuvers may delay the necessity for mask ventilation or intubation while other assessments are ongoing.[32] These teachings are time-honored, but not evidence-based. Bag-valve-mask (BVM) ventilation may be necessary if respirations are deemed insufficient.

Hypoxia should be avoided and oxygen supplementation is routinely recommended, although again outcomes data do not exist. Pulse oximetry may detect unexpected hypoxia and the need for oxygen supplementation. Recently, there have been concerns that hyperoxemia may worsen neuronal injury in post-cardiac-arrest patients. With cardiac resuscitation, there are advocates who suggest maintaining oxygen saturations in the mid 90 percent range by titrating oxygen flow downward if necessary.[31] Application of this to the spinal-cord-injured patient has not been studied.

There is no clear evidence supporting routine endotracheal intubation for patients with a suspected cervical spine injury by EMS providers when the airway is being adequately maintained by the patient or when the airway is improved with BLS maneuvers and adequate respiratory effort is present. Some patients will, however, require emergent or urgent intubation because of associated traumatic injuries or the nature of the spinal cord injury. Patients with high cervical injuries may experience immediate or near-immediate apnea, and may require BVM ventilation with high flow oxygen after opening the airway. There is concern about movement of the cervical spine with these actions and in-line stabilization should be maintained.

Patients with isolated mid-cervical fractures with cord impairment may be communicative and have spontaneous

Table 5.2 Spinal cord levels

Level of spinal cord injury	Resulting loss of function
C3, C4, C5	Diaphragm weakness, respiratory failure
C5	Shrugging of shoulders
C6	Flexion at elbow
C8–T1	Flexion of fingers
L1, L2	Flexion at hip
S1, S2	Plantar flexion of foot
S2, S3, S4	Rectal sphincter tone

respirations, but are at risk from respiratory deterioration. With paralysis of the intercostal muscles from spinal cord injury, the patient becomes dependent on diaphragmatic breathing. The cervical cord segments C-3,4,5 innervate the diaphragm (simple mnemonic – "3,4,5 keeps the diaphragm alive"). Patients may experience fatigue of the diaphragm and progressive respiratory insufficiency; early ventilatory support is recommended[7] (see Table 5.2).

If emergent airway control is needed, current opinion holds that oral intubation with direct laryngoscopy using rapid sequence techniques while maintaining in-line stabilization is safe and effective.[7, 32] Manual in-line stabilization of the cervical spine is recommended during intubation based on trials of uninjured patients, cadavers, retrospective case series and expert opinion. In-line stabilization has not been studied in prospective randomized trials, but data indicate that direct laryngoscopy and intubation are unlikely to cause clinically significant movement of the spine even though manual in-line stabilization may not fully immobilize the cervical spine.[33] In-line stabilization may, however, make direct laryngoscopy more difficult.[32] Video laryngoscopy is rapidly becoming more popular in the emergency setting, and may require less spinal manipulation than direct laryngoscopy.

There is no clear evidence to support the use of any one RSI paralytic agent over another. Succinylcholine remains the agent of choice for rapid sequence intubation in acute spinal-cord-injured patients within the first 48 hours of injury.[7] Propofol, unusual in the prehospital setting, should be used cautiously in the patient with potential hypotension from injuries.

Many other techniques have been advocated, but controlled comparisons are lacking. Supraglottic airway devices, video laryngoscopes, optical stylets and fiber-optic-assisted intubation all have advocates. Intubation with a flexible fiber-optic bronchoscope has been recommended by many as the procedure of choice, but use is limited both by device availability and the necessity for experienced operators.[34] Many of these devices are not yet widely available to the prehospital provider. Prospectively collected evidence is limited and there are no data to suggest better outcomes with any one particular technique.[32] Cricothyroidotomy may be required if the patient cannot be successfully ventilated due to injuries to the pharynx or if orotracheal intubation is unsuccessful. Although obtaining an adequate airway is of paramount importance, providers should be cautious concerning movement of the spine during this procedure.

Blood pressure management

The issue of blood pressure management in spinal-cord-injury patients is complex. In patients with spinal cord injury who are hypotensive, providers should suspect additional traumatic injuries, such as intra-abdominal hemorrhage. As noted above, management of the multi-system trauma patient is controversial. There seems to be general agreement, however, that *profound hypotension should be treated*. For patients with short transport times to a trauma center, judicious fluid management without excessive volume administration has been advocated.

Unrelated to the issue of hypotension caused by traumatic injuries (i.e. hypovolemic shock), patients with spinal cord injury may experience neurogenic shock. This results from the loss of sympathetic tone below the site of the injury. One of the hallmarks of neurogenic shock is hypotension with the absence of tachycardia or even bradycardia, together with the lack of peripheral vasoconstriction typical of hypovolemic shock. Patients are often awake and alert unless there are other associated injuries. *Neurogenic shock is a diagnosis of exclusion*; that is, it should be suspected only after other sources of hypotension, including hemorrhage and cardiac trauma, have been ruled out. Neurogenic shock occurs more frequently in patients with high cervical spinal cord injuries.[35] The misnomer of spinal shock is sometimes applied to this condition, but spinal shock technically describes the loss of reflexes and muscle tone in the acute injury period.

Hypotension worsens traumatic brain injury. Although this concept has been extrapolated to spinal cord injury, convincing data specific to spinal cord injury are lacking.

Two small studies have reported favorable outcomes using fluid and medications in an ICU setting to maintain mean arterial blood pressure (MAP) of 85 mmHg over several days in patients with acute spinal cord injury.[36, 37] Follow-up studies are lacking. Correction of hypotension following acute spinal cord injury is either recommended or regarded as an option in different guidelines.[7, 38] The optimal blood pressure and resuscitation end point for maintenance of spinal cord perfusion are not known. The goal is to maintain tissue perfusion while at the same time avoiding fluid overload.[7] The first step is to restore volume. If volume replacement is corrected and hypotension continues, vasopressors are recommended; again, there is no consensus for a preferred agent.[33, 39] Choices include norepinephrine, phenylephrine, dopamine, dobutamine or epinephrine. Volume expansion and pressors for the patient with an acute cervical spinal cord injury with the goal of maintaining mean arterial blood pressure between 85 and 90 mmHg for seven days is recommended in recent guidelines,[38] although the strength of the recommendation is low and other interpretations of the literature suggest that further studies are needed before this practice is widely implemented.[7] Therapeutic hypothermia has had limited investigation for spinal cord injuries and cannot be advocated at this time.

What is the role of neuroprotective agents for the spinal-cord-injured patient?

There are *currently no neuroprotective agents that have proven effective and beneficial* in patients with acute spinal cord injury.

Few things have been more controversial than the use of steroids. The use of methylprednisolone in acute spinal cord injury was essentially mandated following an NIH-sponsored study that was said to show some minimal benefit to patients with acute spinal cord injury when large doses were administered early.[40] EMS protocols were developed and EMS personnel were involved in giving large doses of steroids by bolus and continuous infusion. Further studies have not borne out any substantial benefit and have found complications with the use of steroids.[41–46] Other reviews and recommendations no longer advocate using steroids for spinal cord injury.[7, 47]

Summary

Given the relatively rare occurrence of spinal cord injuries, it will be difficult to construct prospective clinical trials that will include enough outcomes data to be adequately powered to answer basic questions in the management of the spinal-cord-injured patient. As a consequence, it is likely that treatment recommendations will continue to be based on lower levels of evidence.

Key issues for future investigation

Determining which patients require immobilization

Despite the large amount of published research in this area over the last 15 years, important unsettled questions remain that increase the challenge for EMS providers seeking to apply field assessment protocols.

Selection of spinal assessment criteria

EMS field protocols derived from the NEXUS criteria are not designed to identify 100 percent of patients with a spine injury who require immobilization. While the sensitivity of the NEXUS criteria is quite good, these protocols do not totally eliminate the possibility of not immobilizing a spinal fracture. Studies examining the Canadian C-spine rule have yielded similar sensitivities, but the rule has not been widely adopted by EMS in the United States and is only deployed in a limited fashion in Canada. This may in part arise from the complexity of the rule, as viewed from the perspective of an EMS provider who must make a rapid clinical decision regarding immobilization.[49] For example, the rule requires EMS providers to determine whether an MVC involved speeds in excess of 100 km/hr, but it is often difficult or impossible for providers to know the actual speed. Future studies will hopefully either examine additional or different criteria that are both straightforward to apply and sufficiently sensitive.

Whether to immobilize?

There remains no high-quality published evidence demonstrating that spinal immobilization improves outcomes, even in the context of fractures that are considered to be unstable.[5, 8] In an editorial examining the state of prehospital spinal immobilization, Hauswald argues that "specific treatments that are irrational and which can be safely discarded include the use of backboards for transportation, cervical collar use except in specific injury types, immobilisation of ambulatory patients on backboards, prolonged attempts to stabilise the spine during extrication, mechanical immobilisation of uncooperative or seizing patients and forceful in line stabilisation during airway management."[5] In the absence of data to support changing recommendations, guidelines have retained the traditional practice of full immobilization with modifications to exclude patients with no clinical signs of an acute injury. However, if additional evidence accumulates about harmful effects of immobilization, future guidelines may eliminate or further restrict the use of spinal immobilization. Minimizing spinal movement and pressure on the injured site during EMS care remains a worthwhile and rationale treatment goal, but few options exist other than full immobilization with a rigid cervical collar and long backboard. Vacuum backboards are being employed in some EMS systems and may be a useful option.[5]

In January 2013, the National Association of EMS Physicians and American College of Surgeons Committee on Trauma issued a joint position statement regarding EMS spinal precautions and the use of the long backboard.[50] The position statement recognized that the benefit of long backboards is largely unproven and that the long backboard can induce pain, patient agitation and respiratory compromise, and can decrease tissue perfusion at pressure points, leading to the development of pressure ulcers. The statement urged more judicious use of backboards, and embraced the NEXUS exclusion criteria for avoiding unnecessary immobilization.[50]

The statement also endorsed using a rigid cervical collar and securing the patient firmly to the EMS stretcher as an alternative in some circumstances, including patients found ambulatory at the scene, patients who must be transported for a protracted time and other patients for whom a backboard is not otherwise indicated.

Immobilization in older patients

Studies have noted that spinal assessment protocols may be less sensitive in discerning spinal fractures in older patients (for example, 65 years or older). In these studies, the majority of the patients with spinal fractures who were not immobilized were over 65 years old and most of these fractures were not clinically significant.[2, 11, 12] While excluding older patients from selective immobilization protocols may reduce the incidence of non-immobilized spinal fractures, this benefit must be weighed against the likelihood of increased harm in elderly patients as a consequence of immobilization. It has also been theorized that fractures in older patients may arise from lower energy mechanisms that are less likely to result in clinically significant injuries.[2] Possible age group predisposition to injury merits further study.[2, 11, 12]

Immobilization in children and infants

As noted above, the NEXUS criteria have been found to be reliable in children.[18, 20] However, there were so few cervical spine injuries among the 3,065 children evaluated in the NEXUS study that it was difficult to assess the accuracy of the rule in children with confidence (the 95 percent confidence interval for the sensitivity of the NEXUS criteria for children was 87.8 to 100 percent).[18, 20] More research is needed to determine whether assessment protocols used in adults can be safely applied to younger patients.[12]

Leonard *et al.* found that children who underwent spinal immobilization had a higher degree of pain than children who were not immobilized, and were more likely to undergo radiographic studies and be admitted to the hospital, but were not able to determine if these differences were related to immobilization or to differences in injuries.[51] Recently, there has been increased concern about the amount of radiation to which children are exposed, prompting efforts to reduce radiographic studies where appropriate.[18] More research is needed to assess the management of suspected spine injuries in children, including the applicability of spine assessment protocols, the benefits and disadvantages of spinal immobilization, and techniques for immobilization where warranted.

The question of immobilization of infants (0 to 1 years) has not been examined. In one study, a 9 month old was among the eight patients who had a cervical injury that was missed by the assessment protocol, and the authors suggested that assessment protocols be used with caution in children under age 1.[12] More research is needed.

Non-clinical criteria for selective immobilization

Sochor *et al.* report the development of an entirely new decision rule that does not rely on clinical criteria to make a determination whether to immobilize a patient.[3] In a retrospective analysis of a large national database, the Glass Intact Assures Safe Cervical Spine rule was developed. It was proposed that immobilization is not needed for patients in a motor vehicle crash if:

- patients are between the ages of 16 and 60 years;
- patients were belt-restrained, front-seat occupants;
- there was no airbag deployment; and
- car windows were rolled up and intact.

Prospective validation is required. A non-clinical test, if proven effective, offers the significant advantage of eliminating the ambiguity associated with factors such as "painful, distracting injury."

Blood pressure management

Further studies are needed to define ideal blood pressure management in the patient with acute spinal cord injury and the roles of volume administration and vasopressor use.

REFERENCES

1. Vaillancourt, C., Stiell, I. G., Beaudoin, T. *et al.* (2009). "The out-of-hospital validation of the Canadian C-Spine rule by paramedics," *Ann. Emerg. Med.* 54(5): 672–3.
2. Burton, J. H., Dunn, M. G., Harmon, N. R. *et al.* (2006). "A statewide, prehospital emergency medical service, selective patient spine immobilization protocol," *J. Trauma* 61(1): 161–7.

3. Sochor, M., Althoff, S., Bose, D. *et al.* (2012). "Glass intact assures safe cervical spine protocol," *J. Emerg. Med.*, e-pub, doi: 10.1016/j.jemermed.2012.07.076.

4. Domeier, R. M. Frederiksen, S. M. and Welch, K. (2005). "Prospective performance assessment of an out-of-hospital protocol for selective spine immobilization using clinical spine clearance criteria," *Ann. Emerg. Med.* 46(2): 123–31.

5. Hauswald, M. (2012). "A re-conceptualisation of acute spinal care," *Emerg. Med. J.*, e-pub, PMID: 22962052.

6. Perron, A. D. and Huff, J. S. (2010). "Spinal cord disorders" in J. M. Marx, R. S. Hockberger and R. M. Walls (eds.), *Rosen's Emergency Medicine: Principles and Practice of Emergency Medicine* (Philadelphia, PA: Mosby), pp. 1389–97.

7. Consortium for Spinal Cord Medicine (2008). "Early acute management in adults with spinal cord injury: a clinical practice guideline for health-care professionals," *J. Spinal Cord Med.* 31(4): 408–79.

8. Hauswald, M., Ong, G., Tandberg, D. *et al.* (1998). "Out-of-hospital spinal immobilization: its effect on neurologic injury," *Acad. Emerg. Med.* 5(3): 214–19.

9. Kwan, I., Bunn, F. and Roberts, I. (2001). "Spinal immobilisation for trauma patients," *Cochrane Database Syst. Rev.* 2: CD002803.

10. Haut, E. R., Kalish, B. T., Efron, D. T. *et al.* (2010). "Spine immobilization in penetrating trauma: more harm than good?" *J. Trauma* 68(1): 115–20, discussion 120–1, doi: 10.1097/TA.0b013e3181c9ee58.

11. Myers, L. A., Russi, C. S., Hankins, D. G. *et al.* (2009). "Efficacy and compliance of a prehospital spinal immobilization guideline," *Int. J. Emerg. Med.* 2(1): 13–17.

12. Stroh, G. and Braude, D. (2001). "Can an out-of-hospital cervical spine clearance protocol identify all patients with injuries? An argument for selective immobilization," *Ann. Emerg. Med.* 37(6): 609–15.

13. Hoffman, J. R., Mower, W. R., Wolfson, A. B. *et al.* (2000). "Validity of a set of clinical criteria to rule out injury to the cervical spine in patients with blunt trauma," *N. Engl. J. Med.* 343(2): 94–9.

14. Stiell, I. G., Wells, G. A., Vandemheem, K. L. *et al.* (2001). "The Canadian C-spine rule for radiography in alert and stable trauma patients," *JAMA* 286(15): 1841–8.

15. Stiell, I. G., Clement, C. M., McKnight, D. R. *et al.* (2003). "The Canadian C-spine rule versus the NEXUS Low-Risk Criteria in patients with trauma," *N. Engl. J. Med.* 349(26): 2510–18.

16. Knopp, R. (2004). "Comparing NEXUS and Canadian C-spine decision rules for determining the need for cervical spine radiography," *Ann. Emerg. Med.* 43(4): 518–20.

17. Mower, W. R., Wolfson, A. B., Hoffman, J. R. *et al.* (2004). "The Canadian C-spine rule," *N. Engl. J. Med.* 350(14): 1467–9.

18. Daffner, R. H., Weissman, B. N., Wippold II, F. J. *et al.* (2012). "*Expert Panels on Musculoskeletal and Neurologic Imaging. ACR Appropriateness Criteria° suspected spine trauma*" (online publication) (Reston, VA: American College of Radiology (ACR)).

19. Vaillancourt, C., Charette, M., Kasaboski, A. *et al.* (2011). "Evaluation of the safety of C-spine clearance by paramedics: design and methodology," *BMC Emergency Medicine* 11: 1.

20. Viccello, P., Simon, H., Pressman, B. D. *et al.* (2001). "A prospective multicenter study of cervical spine injury in children," *Pediatrics* 108(2): E20.

21. Theodore, N., Hadley, M. N. and Aarabi, B. (2013). "Guidelines for the management of acute cervical spine and spinal cord injuries," *Neurosurgery* 72(Suppl. 2): 22–34.

22. Baez, A. A. and Schiebel, N. (2006). "Evidence-based emergency medicine/systematic review abstract. Is routine spinal immobilization an effective intervention for trauma patients?" *Ann. Emerg. Med.* 47(1): 110–12.

23. Ahn, H., Nathens, A., MacDonald, R. D. *et al.* (2001). "Pre-hospital care management of a potential spinal cord injured patient: a systematic review of the literature and evidence-based guidelines," *J. Neurotrauma* 28(8): 1341–61.

24. Del Rossi, G., Heffernan, T. P., Horodyski, M. *et al.* (2004). "The effectiveness of extrication collars tested during the execution of spine-board transfer techniques," *Spine J.* 4(6): 619–23.

25. Ben-Galim, P., Dreiangel, N., Mattox, K. L. *et al.* (2010). "Extrication collars can result in abnormal separation between vertebrae in the presence of a dissociative injury," *J. Trauma* 69(2): 447–50.

26. Mobbs, R. J., Stoodley, M. A. and Fuller, J. (2002). "Effect of cervical hard collar on intracranial pressure after head injury," *ANZ J. Surg.* 72(6): 389–91.

27. Hunt, K., Hallworth, S. and Smith, M. (2001). "The effects of rigid collar placement on intracranial and cerebral perfusion pressures," *Anaesthesia* 56(6): 511–13.

28. Del Rossi, G., Rechtine, G. R., Conrad, B. P. *et al.* (2010)."Are scoop stretchers suitable for use on spine-injured patients?" *Am. J. Emerg. Med.* 28(7): 751–6.

29. Shafer, J. S. and Naunheim, R. S. (2009). "Cervical spine motion during extrication: a pilot study," *West J. Emerg. Med.* 10(2): 74–8.

30. Macias, C. A., Rosengart, M. R., Puyana, J. C. *et al.* (2009). "The effects of trauma center care, admission volume, and surgical volume on paralysis after traumatic spinal cord injury," *Ann. Surg.* 249(1): 10–17.

31. Berg, R.A., Hemphill, R., Abella, B. S. *et al.* (2010). "Part 5: Adult Basic Life Support: American Heart Association Guidelines for Cardiopulmonary Resuscitation and Emergency Cardiovascular Care," *Circulation* 122(18 Suppl. 3): S685–705.

32. Ghafoor, A., Martin, T. W., Gopalakrishnan, S. *et al.* (2005). "Caring for patients with cervical spine injuries: what have we learned?" *J. Clin. Anes.* 17(8): 640–9.

33. Manoach, S. and Paladina, L. (2007). "Manual in-line stabilization for acute airway management of suspected cervical spine injury: historical review and current questions," *Ann. Emerg. Med.* 50(3): 236–45.

34. Stein, D. M., Roddy, V., Marx, J. *et al.* (2012). "Emergency neurologic life support: traumatic spine injury," *Neurocrit. Care* 17(Suppl. 1): S102–11.

35. Bilello, J. F., Davis, J. W., Cunningham, M. A. *et al.* (2003). "Cervical spinal cord injury and the need for cardiovascular intervention," *Arch. Surg.* 138(10): 1127–9.

36. Levi, L., Wolf, L. and Belzberg, H. (1993). "Hemodynamic parameters in patients with acute spinal cord trauma: description, intervention, and prediction of outcome," *Neurosurgery* 33(6): 1007–16.

37. Vale, F. L., Burns, J., Jackson, A. B. *et al.* (1997). "Combined medical and surgical treatment after acute spinal cord injury: results of a prospective pilot study to assess the merits of aggressive medical resuscitation and blood pressure management," *J. Neurosurg.* 87(2): 239–46.

38. Ryken, T. C., Hurlbert, R. J., Hadley, M. N. *et al.* (2013). "The acute cardiopulmonary management of patients with cervical cord injuries," *Neurosurgery* 72: S84–92.

39. Stevens, R. D., Bhardwaj, A., Kirsch, J. R. *et al.* (2003). "Critical care and perioperative management in traumatic spinal cord injury," *J. Neurosurg. Anes.* 15: 215–29.

40. Bracken, M. B., Shepard, M. J., Collins, W. F. *et al.* (1990). "A randomized, controlled trial of methylprednisolone or naloxone in the treatment of acute spinal-cord injury – results of the second national acute spinal cord injury study," *N. Engl. J. Med.* 322(20): 1405–11.

41. Levy, M. L., Gans, W., Wijesinghe, H. S. *et al.* (1996). "Use of methylprednisolone as an adjunct in the management of patients with penetrating spinal cord injury: outcome analysis," *Neurosurgery* 39(6): 1141–8.

42. Gerndt, S. J., Rodriguez, J. L., Pawlik, J. W. *et al.* (1997). "Consequences of high-dose steroid therapy for acute spinal cord injury," *J. Trauma* 42(2): 279–84.

43. McCutcheon, E. P., Selassie, A. W., Gu, J. K. *et al.* (2004). "Acute traumatic spinal cord injury, 1993–2000: A population-based assessment of methylprednisolone

administration and hospitalization," *J. Trauma* 56(5): 1076–83.

44. Matsumoto, T., Tamaki, T., Kawakami, M. *et al.* (2001). "Early complications of high-dose methylprednisolone sodium succinate treatment in the follow-up of acute cervical spinal cord injury," *Spine* 26(4): 426–30.

45. Pointillart, V., Petitjean, M. E., Wiart, L. *et al.* (2000). "Pharmacological therapy of spinal cord injury during the acute phase," *Spinal Cord* 38(2): 71–6.

46. Molano Mdel, R., Broton, J. G., Bean, J. A. *et al.* (2002). "Complications associated with the prophylactic use of methylprednisolone during surgical stabilization after spinal cord injury," *J. Neurosurg.* 96(Suppl. 3): 267–72.

47. Chinnock, R. and Roberts, I. (2005). "Gangliosides for acute spinal cord injury," *Cochrane Database Syst. Rev.* 2(2): CD004444.

48. Hurlbert, R. J., Hadley, M. N., Walters, B. C. *et al.* (2013). "Pharmacological therapy for acute spinal cord injury," *Neurosurgery* 72(2): 93–105.

49. Weiner, S. G. (2009). "The actual application of the NEXUS and Canadian C-spine rules by emergency physicians," *Internet J. Emerg. Med.* 5(2), doi: 10.5580/1967.

50. National Association of EMS Physicians and the American College of Surgeons Committee on Trauma (2013). "EMS spinal precautions and the use of the long backboard," *Prehosp. Emerg. Care* 17(3): 392–3.

51. Leonard, J. C., Mao, J. and Jaffe, D. M. (2012). "Potential adverse effects of spinal immobilization in children," *Prehosp. Emerg. Care* 16(4): 513–18.

Chapter 6

Traumatic brain injury

Gregory P. Schaefer and Terry A. Taylor, II

Recommendations

High quality of evidence

No high-quality recommendations may be made based on the available evidence.

Moderate quality of evidence

When EMS professionals skilled and experienced in rapid sequence induction and endotracheal intubation are available, severely brain-injured patients (Glasgow Coma Scale < 9) should receive endotracheal intubation.

Low quality of evidence

1. When pulse oximetry is available, supplemental oxygen should be given as needed to maintain the oxygen saturation above 94 percent. When pulse oximetry is not available, high-flow oxygen should be given.

Prehospital Care of Neurologic Emergencies, ed. Todd J. Crocco and Michael R. Sayre. Published by Cambridge University Press. © Cambridge University Press 2014.

2. When the patient has stable hemodynamic measurements, administration of 1.5 mg/kg of intravenous lidocaine 2 to 3 minutes prior to rapid sequence induction and endotracheal intubation may be considered.

3. In the absence of clinical signs of herniation (for example, unilateral dilated pupil), patients with traumatic brain injury (TBI) should be ventilated to maintain an end-tidal CO_2 value between 30 and 35 mmHg.

4. Crystalloid fluids may be used to support circulation and treat hypotension.

5. Patients with altered mental status following TBI should have immobilization of the cervical spine.

Overview

Traumatic brain injury encompasses a broad spectrum of severity, but these share in common the potential to have a lifetime of impact upon patients. Whether dealing with the athlete sustaining a concussion to the comatose multisystem trauma patient, EMS professionals must be prepared to accurately and quickly assess, treat and transport to the most appropriate facility. The treatment modalities and technologies available to prehospital providers have evolved over the decades and will continue to expand as research continues.

Epidemiology

Annually, 1.5 million patients are treated in US emergency departments for head injury. Among those approximately

52,000 will die of their head injury.[1] Most commonly affected are those less than 30 years of age and those more than 65 years of age. Falls remain the primary mechanism of sustaining a TBI. Interpersonal violence and military conflict are common etiologies among younger victims. TBI results in hospitalization for one-fifth of patients and overall mortality is approximately 3 percent. The financial cost to society, patients and their families related to direct and indirect association with head injury over a lifetime can be overwhelming. As prehospital providers, rapid assessment and appropriate treatment may be able to limit the extent of injury and reduce the lifetime disability.

Anatomy and physiology

The external surface anatomy of the skull is defined by sutures lines that divide the bones – parietal, temporal, frontal and occipital. The skull is of varying thickness and the individual bones become less mobile as ossification occurs in early childhood. Fontanels, non-ossified membranes between the sutures located anteriorly and posteriorly in children, can be important in assessing head-injured infants. A bulging fontanel should raise concern for a severe head injury and possibly elevated intracranial pressure.

The brain is comprised primarily of three major structures: cerebrum, cerebellum and brain stem. Each major structure has many functions and substructures essential for motor and sensory function. When describing lesions or areas of hemorrhage, the overlying bones are used for anatomical reference, i.e. temporal, parietal, etc.

The brain is covered by three layers of tissues with fluid and blood vessels traversing between. The outermost layer, the dura mater, is the toughest. It provides protection to the underlying brain. Several arteries traverse the space between the skull and the dura. Bleeding in this space is known as an epidural hematoma (EDH) and can result in rapid cerebral compression. Bridging veins traverse the space beneath the dura. Injury to the veins results in a subdural hemorrhage (SDH). The arachnoid membrane lies between dura mater and the thinner pia mater. Bleeding beneath this layer is known as a subarachnoid hemorrhage (SAH).

Cerebral perfusion

Due to the high metabolic demand of brain cells, a significant amount of cardiac output is delivered to the brain on a continuous basis. Even short interruptions or decreases in cerebral blood flow (CBF) can result in ischemic injury to the brain.

The brain possesses the ability to autoregulate cerebral blood flow in response to changes in body physiology and metabolic demands within the brain itself. The volume of cerebrospinal fluid within and surrounding the brain may be changed, and blood flow to the brain may be altered by vasoconstriction or vasodilatation. The injured brain may lose the ability to autoregulate. In this case, cerebral blood flow is regulated only by cardiac output and circulating blood volume.

Prehospital providers may clinically notice inadequate cerebral blood flow manifesting as changes in mental status or seizure activity.

Absent a form of shock, the foremost etiology of inadequate cerebral blood flow is elevated intracranial pressure (ICP). The intracranial volume is fixed and occupied predominantly by brain parenchyma, cerebrospinal fluid and blood. When additional material is introduced into this space or the volume of that space is reduced, the pressure in that space (ICP) increases. In the absence of autoregulation, the body has limited compensatory mechanisms, all of which are deleterious in the end. Clinically, the prehospital provider may witness Cushing reflex: irregularity of the respiratory pattern, a widening of pulse pressure and bradycardia. This is a physiologic effort to reduce cerebral blood flow to decrease ICP. In blunt trauma without open skull fracture, the brainstem will herniate through the foramen magnum at the base of the skull. Herniation effectively reduces the intracranial volume and pressure, but results in loss of blood flow to the brainstem. Prolonged and untreated herniation may progress to brain death.

Assessment

TBI may occur as an isolated injury or in the context of multisystem trauma. Prehospital providers must remain cognizant of the need to prevent secondary brain injury within the context of treating the entire patient. Untreated exsanguination, airway compromise or ineffective breathing can contribute to ongoing secondary brain injury.

A brief neurologic examination that can be quickly repeated and achieves consistent results between examiners is necessary. The Glasgow Coma Scale (GCS) was first published in 1974.[2] The score consists of three subgroup assessments and associated "scores" based upon level of consciousness: Eye Opening (1–4), Verbal Response (1–5) and Motor Response (1–6). Scores range from 3 to 15. Despite widespread use, recent studies have raised doubts regarding inter-rater variability and the challenges faced by providers when using it.

The GCS motor response score appears to have the greatest value in terms of predicting injury severity and outcome. This value must be assessed within the context of the patient's ability to have a motor response when affected by chemical paralysis, pain, fracture or spinal cord injury. Several newer, more simplified scales to assess the level of consciousness have been developed and validated. These scores have not been widely implemented; however, further comparison with the GCS could yield interesting results.

Another element of the neurological exam assessed during a primary survey is an assessment of the pupils. Pupillary size and reactivity to light should be quickly assessed. Presence of a markedly dilated or "blown" pupil may be a sign of severe head injury with rising intracranial pressure. Unreactive and bilaterally dilated pupils portend a worse prognosis. The above findings can also be associated with isolated optic nerve injury or administration of an anticholinergic such as atropine.

During the secondary survey, a more comprehensive physical examination of the head and face may reveal skull fractures, drainage of cerebrospinal fluid from the nose or ears, or exposed brain matter. A rapid yet thorough assessment to identify motor or sensory deficits should be undertaken. Throughout the treatment and transport, neurologic function should be reassessed frequently.

Injury classification

A. Mild traumatic brain injury (GCS 13–15)
   1. most common;
   2. awareness increasing that concussion is a form of TBI;
   3. may or may not have loss of consciousness;
   4. up to one-third will have intracranial hemorrhage;
   5. typically do well; however, post-concussive symptoms may persist;
   6. mortality < 1 percent.
B. Moderate traumatic brain injury (GCS 9–12)
   1. transient or persistent confusion;
   2. mortality 5 percent;
   3. if not identified or treated properly, may progress to severe brain injury;
   4. concern for missed spinal cord or musculoskeletal injury due to degree of altered mental status.
C. Severe traumatic brain injury (GCS ≤ 8)
   1. mortality > 20 percent, may be higher without appropriate treatment;
   2. high suspicion for other severe injury;
   3. prevention of secondary injury critical to reduce morbidity and mortality;
   4. potential for airway compromise.

Primary brain injury

Primary injury occurs at the time of initial trauma, whether by a blunt or penetrating mechanism. Treatment options are non-existent. Direct forces occur from direct impact to the head. These forces can result in skull fractures and cerebral contusions. Prevention of these primary injuries can be achieved through proper athletic techniques or properly fitted protective gear (e.g. helmets).

Acceleration/deceleration forces occur with rapid changes in velocity. When a vehicle collides, the patient and the patient's brain are travelling at the same velocity; however, the rate of deceleration may be different due to safety equipment. When the brain decelerates at a different velocity relative to the skull, contusion may result from abrupt contact with the inner surface of the skull. Further, epidural arteries and subdural veins may be torn during this process. In the elderly, simple ground-level falls may produce enough force to result in these types of injuries.

Shearing forces result from glancing blows. This commonly occurs in motor vehicle collisions that are not direct impact or in athletic events. The rotational forces can yield injury to the nerve sheaths at a microscopic level. While CT imaging may not be impressive due to the nature of the injury, the extent of this injury may have long-term and catastrophic consequences.

The EMS professional has the opportunity to participate in prevention. Presentations to schools, youth sports organizations and in public forums are methods to share information about safe behaviors and use of safety equipment. Several organizations and government entities have resources to facilitate public education. The Centers for Disease Control and Prevention offer a "Heads Up" program to educate youth and adults regarding sports-related head injury.[3] Some literature supports educational efforts being aimed at children as they may be more willing to implement changes in behavior.

An accurate report on the exact mechanism of injury is helpful to trauma center staff. Documentation may be enhanced with diagrams, photos and, in some sporting events, video replays.

Secondary brain injury

A complex series of cellular and molecular events occur after the primary brain injury. As a direct result of the injury and from secondary effects, nerve cell death will transpire over the ensuing minutes, hours and days. Unfortunately, this process can lead to a self-propagating cycle, which left unbroken can result in severe neurologic damage or death. While specific processes are not visible to EMS professionals, they have the ability to break the cycle and improve outcomes by addressing secondary brain insults, such as hypotension, hypoxia, severe acid–base derangements, hypoglycemia, fever and seizure activity.

Whether trauma, stroke or other acute neurologic emergency, neurologic damage occurs as a result of ongoing hypoperfusion to the brain. Brain cells are particularly sensitive to hypoxia. Hypoperfusion can be multifactorial, but is clinically manifested as hypotension and hypoxia. Even a single episode of hypotension may have a significant detrimental effect on the injured brain.[4] A larger and more contemporary meta-analysis of 8,721 patients (IMPACT study) further confirmed that hypotension and hypoxia were significantly associated with poor outcomes when measured at a 6-month interval.[5] Hypoxia itself is also associated with worsened outcomes.[6]

A post-hoc analysis of 81 trauma patients sustaining severe TBI and having a combined transport time and emergency department stay of less than 2 hours evaluated the impact of secondary brain insult on several outcome variables.[7] Hypocapnea (low PCO_2), hypotension and acidosis were the most commonly identified insults. The three factors associated with worst outcome (i.e. severe morbidity and mortality) were hypotension (68 percent), hyperglycemia (40 percent) and hypothermia (26 percent).

Hypotension

Guidelines for the triage and treatment of brain-injured patients have long identified blood pressure as a prominent criterion. EMS professionals practice in environments that are often austere and noisy. Automated non-invasive blood pressure (NIBP) monitoring of critically ill patients may provide readings that are inaccurate.[8] Patient movement, road noise or turbulence, and use of inappropriately sized cuffs, can adversely affect NIBP accuracy. If automated NIBP monitoring is used, the readings should be correlated regularly with a manually obtained blood pressure.

The number of hypotensive episodes also carries increased risk for TBI patients. In one study, severely multisystem-injured patients with severe TBI (median GCS of 7) sustained at least one episode of hypotension in 24 percent of cases.[9] Among this subgroup, the mortality rate was 65 percent. When two or more episodes of hypotension occurred, the risk of morality, compared to patients without hypotension, increased dramatically.[9]

Global hypoxia

Hypoxia has a detrimental impact on the outcome of TBI patients. Among 150 patients transported by helicopter with continuous pulse oximetry, isolated hypoxia ($SPO_2 < 90$ percent with normal blood pressure) occurred in 25 percent, and hypoxia with hypotension occurred in 4 percent. Isolated hypoxia increased mortality from 20 to 37 percent. Multivariate analysis found prehospital hypoxia to increase mortality risk by 2.6 times baseline.[10]

Acid–base derangements

Acidosis in trauma patients generally indicates inadequate perfusion, most commonly related to hemorrhagic shock. Clearance of acidosis, indicating effective resuscitation, has been correlated with improved outcomes. Acidosis has a protective effect in that it increases oxygen delivery to tissues by altering the function of hemoglobin. Conversely, acidosis may inhibit normal clotting function.

When cells do not receive a sufficient supply of oxygen to sustain their need for energy, anaerobic metabolism increases and produces lactate (an acid). The lactate accumulates in the serum until it is cleared by the liver and other tissues. In essence, lactate levels are a measure of "oxygen debt." Prehospital measurement of lactate is feasible and identifies patients with significant injury earlier than measurement of an abnormal pulse rate or blood pressure.[11]

Blood glucose derangements

Aberrations in serum blood sugar, both hypoglycemia and hyperglycemia, especially if untreated or sustained, may negatively impact on the outcome of TBI patients. Hyperglycemia is a common finding among severely injured patients due to the stress response. The physiologic impact of hyperglycemia on the brain is complex. In the OPTIMISM trial, 213 patients with moderate to severe TBI were evaluated for complications that occurred after admission to the ICU.[12] Hyperglycemia occurred in 83 percent of the subjects, and mortality was more than doubled. Yet, aggressive treatment of hyperglycemia may not improve neurological outcome because insulin treatment increases the risk of hypoglycemia, which has been associated with worse outcomes among other groups of critically ill patients.[13]

Isolated head injury and hypoglycemia share many clinical manifestations. The paramedic should check blood glucose in patients with altered mental status. More than one patient has been cured of focal neurological deficits with intravenous dextrose administration for a blood glucose level of less than 60 mg/dL.

Targeted temperature management

Hypothermia in TBI patients can be a significant challenge for all providers. Multisystem trauma patients fare worse when hypothermia is present. Conversely, therapeutic hypothermia has been explored as a treatment for patients sustaining cardiac arrest, spinal cord injury and traumatic brain injury.

A meta-analysis of 12 studies among over 1,300 patients reviewed the impact of short-term and long-term cooling protocols on neurologic outcome among TBI patients. Only the long-term or goal-directed protocols demonstrated a benefit in regard to mortality and improved neurologic outcome. The maximum benefit seemed to occur when cooling began early, continued for > 72 hours, and targeted a core temperature between 32 and 34 °C.[14] At present, there is insufficient evidence to recommend for or against routine use of targeted temperature management for TBI.[15]

Seizures

The occurrence of early seizure post-TBI is approximately 2 percent based upon series from the 1980s and 1990s.

Severe TBI patients experience seizures more frequently. EMS professionals should treat ongoing seizures in patients with TBI just like other patients with seizures. See Chapter 3 on seizures for more information.

Key challenges

Despite the tireless efforts made by authors of the second edition of the "Brain Trauma Foundation Guidelines for the Prehospital Treatment of Traumatic Brain Injury," every recommendation is classified as "Weak based upon Level III evidence," which, at best, are poorly designed randomized control trials.[1]

Endotracheal intubation

When EMS professionals skilled and experienced in rapid sequence induction and endotracheal intubation are available, severely brain-injured patients (Glasgow Coma Scale < 9) should receive endotracheal intubation (moderate quality of evidence).

The decision to manage the airway of the TBI patient is challenging. For patients with severe TBI, endotracheal intubation is the most common method of establishing a definitive airway, i.e. a cuffed tube within the trachea. The benefits of endotracheal intubation include limiting aspiration of gastric contents, improving control over oxygenation and ventilation, and facilitating administration of sedative, analgesic and paralytic drugs for enhanced patient comfort and safety. Yet, the procedure itself has the risk of disability and death.

The question is whether severely brain-injured patients benefit from endotracheal intubation prior to hospital arrival. Perhaps the key determinant is the skill set of the available EMS professionals. Highly trained and experienced paramedics can safely and effectively use rapid sequence induction (RSI) and endotracheal intubation to manage severe TBI prior to hospital arrival.

RSI and intubation are different procedures. Drug administration is the core of RSI, with the goal of quickly inducing unconsciousness and relaxation to facilitate performance of endotracheal intubation. Typically, sedatives and neuromuscular blocking agents with a short time of onset and duration are given intravenously. Commonly, RSI is a tightly controlled procedure performed by experienced field providers who have been trained with 40 to 50 mentored procedures in the operating suite and field environments.[16] RSI use should be subject to review for improvement opportunities.

In one busy helicopter EMS system where paramedics regularly performed prehospital rapid sequence induction (RSI) under the watchful eye of a performance improvement process, major trauma patients were treated with RSI using neuromuscular blocking agents and general anesthetics followed by endotracheal intubation.[17] Among 175 patients, 88% of whom had at least moderate head injuries, 97% were intubated successfully. Complications were infrequent, and no esophageal intubations occurred. In comparison to patients who were not intubated, RSI and intubation added an average of only 6 minutes to on-scene time.[17]

A randomized trial assigned 312 severely brain-injured adults to either prehospital rapid sequence intubation by experienced paramedics or transport of patients to a hospital emergency department for intubation by physicians.[18] The success rate for the paramedic RSI-assisted intubation was 97 percent and increased the rate of favorable neurological outcome at 6 months compared to intubation after hospital arrival.[18]

When highly trained and experienced EMS professionals are not readily available, then other options may be preferable since observational data suggests that attempting endotracheal intubation could be harmful.[19] Less invasive airway adjuncts (for example, nasopharyngeal or oropharyngeal airways) together with high-flow oxygen may be used without administration of paralytic drugs. Often, these patients can be successfully oxygenated, some may also need assisted ventilation with a bag-valve mask system, while being transported to the emergency department for a physician to perform RSI and endotracheal intubation.

Lidocaine use during RSI

When the patient has stable hemodynamic measurements, administration of 1.5 mg/kg of intravenous lidocaine 2 to 3 minutes prior to rapid sequence induction and endotracheal intubation may be considered (low quality of evidence).

In animals with experimentally created intracranial hypertension, the intravenous administration of lidocaine reduces intracranial pressure.[20] Interestingly, both lidocaine and cocaine were associated with neuroprotection among head-injured animals.[21]

Laryngoscopy and intubation are procedures that have been associated with an increase in sympathetic nervous system tone and intracranial pressure. The premise of lidocaine premedication is to blunt this effect. Endotracheal lidocaine prevented elevation in ICP associated with airway suctioning.[22]

When used, lidocaine administration to prevent ICP elevation during intubation is typically done in the following manner: 1.5 mg/kg administered intravenously 2 to 3 minutes prior to laryngoscopy.

Oxygenation

When pulse oximetry is available, supplemental oxygen should be given as needed to maintain the oxygen saturation above 94 percent. When pulse oximetry is not available, high-flow oxygen should be given (low quality of evidence).

An appropriate amount of oxygen should be provided to avoid hypoxia at all times. In the event that pulse oximetry is available, adjusting the oxygen flow to achieve oxygen saturations > 94 percent is desirable. Some might argue for a different threshold value of oxygen saturation. There is no evidence that a particular oxygen saturation value results in improved clinical outcomes compared with a different value, as long as the values are at least 90 percent. However, there is evidence that hypoxia, even transient hypoxia, is harmful.[6] There is limited evidence that extreme hyperoxia (> 500 mmHg) is also harmful.[6] Thus, a strategy of guiding oxygen administration using pulse oximetry is attractive. Nonetheless, there are no human trials of different oxygen administration strategies for patients with TBI.

Ventilation

In the absence of clinical signs of herniation (for example, unilateral dilated pupil), patients with TBI should be ventilated to maintain an end-tidal CO_2 value between 30 and 35 mmHg (low quality of evidence).

Decreasing the concentration of carbon dioxide (CO_2) in the blood below normal values causes cerebral vasoconstriction, reducing the cerebral blood volume and flow. This may have a temporary benefit by reducing intracranial pressure (ICP) in the setting of impending herniation of brain contents through the tentorium. Conversely, when the vasoconstriction is prolonged, a state of cerebral hypoperfusion can exist, resulting in ischemia-related injury. Many TBI patients who are intubated and hand ventilated develop a hyperventilation-associated respiratory alkalosis. With the availability of continuous capnography in the prehospital setting, EMS professionals can monitor the effect of their ventilations and adjust rate and tidal volume.

A study of 574 trauma patients intubated in the prehospital setting evaluated the frequency of ventilatory derangements.[23] About 18 percent of all patients were hyperventilated resulting in a $pCO_2 < 30$ mmHg on trauma center arrival. Patients who maintained pCO_2 within the target range of 30 to 35 mmHg had improved outcomes, inclusive of those with isolated TBI.[23] Others found similar results in different cities.[24]

Since few prehospital providers have access to arterial blood gas analysis, end-tidal CO_2 measurement offers the promise of monitoring ventilation and achieving the goal arterial concentration. Yet end-tidal CO_2 measurement may not provide a close correlation for arterial CO_2 measurement in major trauma patients due to concomitant lung injury or tissue hypoperfusion.[25] Targeting an end-tidal CO_2 value of about 35 ± 5 mmHg results in the arterial pCO_2 in the goal range only about 38 percent of the time.

If end-tidal CO_2 monitoring is not available, the initial ventilation rate should be:

Adults and adolescents (age > 14):	10 breaths/min
Children (age 2–14):	20 breaths/min
Infants (birth–24 months):	25 breaths/min

Resuscitation fluids

Crystalloid fluids may be used to support circulation and treat hypotension.

Hypotension is associated with adverse outcomes for patients with TBI. Most EMS systems use isotonic fluids for the resuscitation of TBI patients, and millions of liters of such fluids have been given to patients. Yet there is little evidence to guide the amount or specific composition of the resuscitation fluid.[26] Limited evidence suggests that there may be an advantage to lactated Ringer's solution compared to normal saline.[27]

A large multicenter trial conducted by the Resuscitation Outcomes Consortium evaluated the role of hypertonic saline (HTS) $\pm$ dextran versus isotonic fluids for the treatment of TBI patients.[28] The trial was discontinued for futility after randomizing 1,331 patients without a hint of benefit.

Coexisting spine injuries

Patients with altered mental status following traumatic brain injury should have immobilization of the cervical spine.

A review of patients admitted to a large spinal cord injury rehabilitation institute indicates that 60 percent of SCI patients suffered from some degree of TBI concurrently.[29] Due to the alteration in mental status associated with TBI, symptoms such as neck pain, which would otherwise suggest spine injury, may not be apparent. Application of a rigid cervical immobilization collar is prudent. Cervical collars can increase intracranial pressure and should be appropriately sized to mitigate this effect.[30]

Summary

- recognize the signs and symptoms of brain injury ranging from mild to severe;
- never underestimate the severity of brain injury based upon your first interaction with a patient;

- be proactive within your community to prevent primary brain injury;
- quickly identify and treat signs that could contribute to secondary brain insult; and
- rapidly transport TBI patients to the most appropriate trauma center.

Traumatic brain injury is too often an unrecognized disease. The consequences of ineffective, untimely and inadequate treatment can have a devastating impact on the lives of our patients. Astute EMS professionals will possess the knowledge of anatomy, physiology and pathophysiology to recognize and appropriately treat brain-injured patients. While the duration of your contact with patients may be limited relative to the time they are treated and the need for recovery, the impact of your skills may last a lifetime.

Key issues for future investigation

- What is the best fluid for resuscitation of the patient with traumatic brain injury?
- What is the best airway and ventilation strategy in the prehospital setting for treatment of TBI?

REFERENCES

1. Brain Trauma Foundation (2013). "TBI statistics," available at www.braintrauma.org/tbi-faqs/tbi-statistics.
2. Teasdale, G. and Jennett, B. (1974). "Assessment of coma and impaired consciousness. A practical scale," *Lancet* 2(7872): 81–4.

3. Centers for Disease Control and Prevention (CDC) (2013). "Heads up: concussion in youth sports," available at www.cdc.gov/concussion/HeadsUp/youth.html.

4. Chesnut, R. M., Marshall, L. F., Klauber, M. R. *et al.* (1993). "The role of secondary brain injury in determining outcome from severe head injury," *J. Trauma* 34(2): 216–22.

5. McHugh, G. S., Engel, D. C., Butcher, I. *et al.* (2007). "Prognostic value of secondary insults in traumatic brain injury: results from the IMPACT study," *J. Neurotrauma* 24(2): 287–93.

6. Davis, D. P., Meade, W., Sise, M. J. *et al.* (2009). "Both hypoxemia and extreme hyperoxemia may be detrimental in patients with severe traumatic brain injury," *J. Neurotrauma* 26(12): 2217–23.

7. Jeremitsky, E., Omert, L., Dunham, C. M. *et al.* (2003). "Harbingers of poor outcome the day after severe brain injury: hypothermia, hypoxia, and hypoperfusion," *J. Trauma* 54(2): 312–19.

8. Davis, J. W., Davis, I. C., Bennink, L. D. *et al.* (2003). "Are automated blood pressure measurements accurate in trauma patients?" *J. Trauma* 55(5): 860–3.

9. Manley, G., Knudson, M. M., Morabito, D. *et al.* (2001). "Hypotension, hypoxia, and head injury: frequency, duration, and consequences," *Arch. Surgery* 136(10): 1118–23.

10. Chi, J. H., Knudson, M. M., Vassar, M. J. *et al.* (2006). "Prehospital hypoxia affects outcome in patients with traumatic brain injury: a prospective multicenter study," *J. Trauma* 61(5): 1134–41.

11. Guyett, F. (2012). *Biomarker Lactate for Assessment of Shock in Trauma* (Los Angeles, CA: Resuscitation Science Symposium).

12. Muehlschlegel, S., Carandang, R., Ouillette, C. *et al.* (2013). "Frequency and impact of intensive care unit complications on moderate-severe traumatic brain injury: early results of the Outcome Prognostication in Traumatic Brain Injury (OPTIMISM) Study," *Neurocrit. Care* 18(3): 318–31.

13. Kramer, A., Roberts, D. and Zygun, D. (2012). "Optimal glycemic control in neurocritical care patients: a systematic review and meta-analysis," *Crit. Care* 16(5): R203.

14. Fox, J. L., Vu, E. N., Doyle-Waters, M. *et al.* (2010). "Prophylactic hypothermia for traumatic brain injury: a quantitative systematic review," *CJEM* 12(4): 355–64.

15. Nunnally, M., Jaeschke, R., Bellingan, G. *et al.* (2011). "Targeted temperature management in critical care: a report and recommendations from five professional societies," *Crit. Care Med.* 39(5): 1113–25.

16. Warner, K., Carlbom, D., Cooke, C. *et al.* (2010). "Paramedic training for proficient prehospital endotracheal intubation," *Prehosp. Emerg. Care* 14(1): 103–8.

17. Fakhry, S. M., Scanlon, J. M., Robinson, L. *et al.* (2006). "Prehospital rapid sequence intubation for head trauma: conditions for a successful program," *J. Trauma* 60(5): 997–1001.

18. Bernard, S., Nguyen, V., Cameron, P. *et al.* (2010). "Prehospital rapid sequence intubation improves

functional outcome for patients with severe traumatic brain injury: a randomized controlled trial," *Ann. Surg.* 252(6): 959–65.

19. Wang, H., Brown, S., Macdonald, R. *et al.* (2014). "Association of out-of-hospital advanced airway management with outcomes after traumatic brain injury and hemorrhagic shock in the ROC hypertonic saline trial," *Emerg. Med. J.* 31(3): 186–91.

20. Evans, D. E. and Kobrine, A. I. (1987). "Reduction of experimental intracranial hypertension by lidocaine," *Neurosurgery* 20(4): 542–7.

21. Muir, J. K., Lyeth, B. G., Hamm, R. J. *et al.* (1995). "The effect of acute cocaine or lidocaine on behavioral function following fluid percussion brain injury in rats," *J. Neurotrauma* 12(1): 87–97.

22. Bilotta, F., Branca, G., Lam, A. *et al.* (2008). "Endotracheal lidocaine in preventing endotracheal suctioning-induced changes in cerebral hemodynamics in patients with severe head trauma," *Neurocrit. Care* 8(2): 241–6.

23. Warner, K. J., Cuschieri, J., Copass, M. K. *et al.* (2007). "The impact of prehospital ventilation on outcome after severe traumatic brain injury," *J. Trauma* 62(6): 1330–6, discussion 6–8.

24. Davis, D., Peay, J., Sise, M. *et al.* (2010). "Prehospital airway and ventilation management: a trauma score and injury severity score-based analysis," *J. Trauma* 69(2): 294–301.

25. Warner, K., Cuschieri, J., Garland, B. *et al.* (2009). "The utility of early end-tidal capnography in monitoring

ventilation status after severe injury," *J. Trauma* 66(1): 26–31.

26. Myburgh, J. and Mythen, M. (2013). "Resuscitation fluids," *N. Engl. J. Med.* 369(13): 1243–51.

27. Handy, J. and Soni, N. (2008). "Physiological effects of hyperchloraemia and acidosis," *Br. J. Anaesth.* 101(2): 141–50.

28. Bulger, E., May, S., Brasel, K. *et al.* (2010). "Out-of-hospital hypertonic resuscitation following severe traumatic brain injury: a randomized controlled trial," *JAMA* 304(13): 1455–64.

29. Macciocchi, S., Seel, R., Thompson, N. *et al.* (2008). "Spinal cord injury and co-occurring traumatic brain injury: assessment and incidence," *Arch. Phys. Med. Rehabil.* 89(7): 1350–7.

30. Dunham, C., Carter, K., Castro, F. *et al.* (2011). "Impact of cervical spine management brain injury on functional survival outcomes in comatose, blunt trauma patients with extremity movement and negative cervical spine CT: application of the Monte Carlo simulation," *J. Neurotrauma* 28(6): 1009–19.

Chapter 7

Altered mental status

Hollynn Larrabee and Leslie A. Willard

Recommendations

High quality

There are insufficient data to support high quality recommendations for this topic.

Moderate quality

1. In adult and pediatric patients with altered mental status, emergent treatments including airway stabilization, glucose and naloxone administration should be considered prior to transport.
2. Emergent tracheal intubation:
   (a) Nasotracheal intubation should not be performed in the prehospital setting regardless of the level of training of the prehospital provider.
   (b) Prehospital providers should be aware of lower intubation success rates for patients in the following

Prehospital Care of Neurologic Emergencies, ed. Todd J. Crocco and Michael R. Sayre. Published by Cambridge University Press. © Cambridge University Press 2014.

subcategories: trauma, non-arrest and pediatrics. It is prudent to consider other airway management and ventilation techniques, including bag-valve-mask and the placement of a rescue airway device, given high rates of unsuccessful attempts even with appropriate pharmacologic agents.

(c) Prehospital care providers must establish a safe airway with adequate ventilation in patients with respiratory or ventilatory failure; this may or may not be a definitive tracheal airway.

3. Administration of glucose:

(a) If IV access can be obtained, glucose remains the preferred treatment of hypoglycemia, with IM glucagon being given if an IV is unobtainable.

4. Route of naloxone administration:

(a) In hemodynamically stable patients with spontaneous respirations, intranasal naloxone is the preferred route over intramuscular or intravenous given equal efficacy and increased provider safety.

Low quality

1. Emergent endotracheal intubation:

(a) Intubation for patients with a GCS < 8 may not be necessary except in cases of obvious airway compromise (severe stroke, respiratory failure or cardiac arrest).

(b) Prehospital providers should be aware that studies predict that the most difficult intubations are in patients

with a GCS of between 7 and 9 and have backup and
adjunct devices prepared.

2. Safety of non-transport in insulin-dependent diabetes
   mellitus (IDDM) patients after receiving glucose for
   hypoglycemia:
   (a) If blood sugar has returned to normal and the patient
       has decision-making capacity, it is safe to not transport.

3. Empiric use of naloxone in patients with altered mental
   status (AMS):
   (a) The empiric use of naloxone in all patients with altered
       mental status is not justified. Naloxone use should be
       limited to patients with suspected opiate overdose or
       patients with AMS and less than 12 respirations per
       minute.

4. There were no studies in these areas specific to pediatric
   patients.

Overview

Prehospital care providers frequently encounter patients with
altered mental status (AMS). One of the more difficult aspects
of managing these patients is assessing the extensive
differential etiology of the symptoms. Altered mental status
can broadly be separated into traumatic and non-traumatic
causes, with non-traumatic causes being the focus of this
chapter.

Obtaining a brief history and performing a primary
assessment are key factors in determining the cause of the

patient's inability to respond appropriately. A more thorough assessment, although important, should be deferred until any potential life threats are identified and treated. Whether the cause is hypoglycemia, drug overdose or a traumatic incident, quick action by the prehospital care provider is imperative. Durant and Sporer[1] conducted a large cross-sectional review of prehospital care records and discovered that 27 percent of all prehospital patients had some altered level of consciousness. The study found that diabetic patients were the most common group to present as altered and most likely to present with a severely abnormal GCS. Known medical conditions most prominently associated with altered mental status included history of seizures, alcohol use, stroke/TIA, diabetes and other substance abuse.

Initially when encountering an altered patient, prehospital care providers must focus on assessment of airway, breathing and circulation, as well as initial stabilization. Once ABCs are stable, obtaining blood glucose early in the assessment process is critical. Due to the short- and long-term sequelae of hypoglycemia, correcting hypoglycemia early can decrease morbidity and mortality, especially in cardiac and stroke patients.[2] Finally, a comprehensive history should be obtained whenever possible. Prehospital care providers should focus on history of current symptoms, past medical history including similar prior episodes, changes in medications and substance abuse, including looking for drug paraphernalia at the scene. In addition, the mnemonic AEIOUTIPS is frequently used in the prehospital setting to help formulate a differential diagnosis for patients with altered mental status.

A	Alcohol, abuse of substances
E	Epilepsy, electrolyte abnormalities, endocrine disorders
I	Insulin
O	Overdose, oxygen deficiency
U	Uremia
T	Trauma, temperature abnormality, tumor
I	Infection
P	Poisoning, psychiatric conditions
S	Shock, stroke

Prehospital treatment in patients with altered mental status has long been an area of controversy. Actions range from obtaining a blood glucose reading to advanced airway management. Interventions such as administration of glucose to hypoglycemic patients or administration of naloxone to assist with respiratory management of suspected opiate overdoses should be done early. The appropriateness of prehospital intubation has been particularly controversial. This likely reflects the large variation of skill level and procedural experience of prehospital care providers when correlated with successful attempts. Many studies have been done to evaluate the efficacy of prehospital emergency intubation. Intubating all patients with a GCS < 8 may not be necessary. Evaluation of each patient, circumstances of their current condition and likely ability to maintain a patent airway must guide the prehospital provider in making the decision to intubate.

The pediatric altered patient is especially challenging. AMS in the child may present as irritability, decreased interaction or complete unresponsiveness. The causes of altered mental status in children are numerous. The AEIOUTIPS mnemonic is useful here as well, but must be expanded with additional causes unique to pediatric patients. While not exhaustive, this list includes abuse (non-accidental trauma), encephalopathy, inborn errors of metabolism and intussusception.[3] As with adults, altered mental status in children is secondary to an underlying cause. Performing a focused assessment, obtaining a pertinent history, establishing a differential diagnosis and providing appropriate interventions should be performed in a systematic fashion.

Prehospital providers must always approach the management of the patient with an altered mental status in a systematic fashion and with attention to detail. Interventions and procedures to evaluate and treat the patient need to be performed simultaneously. Primary attention needs to be given to reversing those conditions that can be treated in the field, maintaining an open airway and supporting vital signs.

Key challenges

Studies on the efficacy of prehospital intubation

1. Nasotracheal intubation should not be performed in the prehospital setting regardless of the level of training of the prehospital provider.
2. Prehospital providers should be aware of lower intubation success rates for patients in the following subcategories: trauma, non-arrest and pediatrics. It is prudent to consider other airway management and ventilation techniques,

including bag-valve-mask and the placement of a rescue airway device given high rates of unsuccessful attempts even with appropriate pharmacologic agents.

3. Prehospital care providers must establish a safe airway with adequate ventilation in patients with respiratory or ventilatory failure; this may or may not be a definitive tracheal airway.

Prehospital endotracheal intubation has been performed in the United States for over 30 years, but has been the source of considerable debate for the past 10 years.[4, 5] This is primarily due to the large variance of reported success rates in multiple studies of both adult and pediatric patients[6, 7, 8] and the negative outcome associated with the inability to successfully intubate the patient in the field.[9, 10]

In a comprehensive meta-analysis of over 350 scientific articles, Hubble *et al.*[4] systematically reviewed the literature regarding prehospital non-physician intubation success rates. The authors found that the overall rate of intubation success was 86.3 percent by non-physician clinicians. Stated another way, this represents one failed airway in seven attempts. Pediatric studies alone revealed a lower success rate of 83.2 percent. Significantly, the study found much higher success rates in non-trauma patients (88.6 vs. 73.7 percent in trauma patients) and patients in cardiac arrest (91.2 vs. 70.4 percent in non-arrest patients). When evaluating methods of intubation as a subset, rapid sequence intubation (RSI) with direct visualization was the most successful method (96.7 percent). This highlights the difficulty of intubating non-arrest patients without sedation and neuromuscular blockade. Nasotracheal intubation was the least successful technique, with only 73.1 percent success. Of note, even when including prehospital physicians in the pooled data set, nasotracheal intubation success rate remained low at 75.9 percent, suggesting that this is an inappropriate method for intubation in the prehospital setting regardless of provider training level.

A Cochrane review of "Emergency intubation for acutely ill and injured patients"[11] further evaluated three randomized controlled trials (RCTs) to assess the efficacy of intubation in the prehospital environment compared to alternative airway management. The authors concluded that the efficacy of prehospital emergent endotracheal intubation has still not been rigorously studied given the current paucity of high quality data. They surmised that the skill of the operator might be the key determinant of efficacy, regardless of patient factors, given markedly lower success rates in paramedics compared to physicians.

More recently, Lossius *et al.*[12] conducted a large meta-analysis of 58 studies that compared intubation success rates between physicians and non-physicians in the prehospital setting. The success rate of physicians was 99 percent compared to 85 percent in non-physicians. This trend remained true even when sedation and neuromuscular blockade were available to non-physicians with 5 percent of apneic patients with an unsecured airway. The article concludes that prehospital systems with non-physicians should concentrate on basic and advanced airway techniques other than endotracheal intubation for patient safety.

Finally, Wang *et al.*[13] used a multivariate analysis of prospectively derived data to identify situations prone to prehospital intubation failure. The goal of this study was to help providers identify high risk, difficult airways proactively based on initial focused assessment where alternative airway management may be more effective. Patients at highest risk of prehospital intubation failure included those with the presence of clenched jaw/trismus, intact gag reflex or increased weight. Interestingly, those patients who had either IV access or electrocardiogram (ECG) prior to intubation attempts were also at a high risk of failure, which the authors believe was due to these scenarios functioning as surrogate markers for non-cardiac-arrest patients with less emergent need for intubation.

Studies on efficacy of glucose administration

If IV access can be obtained, glucose remains the preferred treatment of hypoglycemia with IM glucagon being given if an IV is unobtainable.

Hypoglycemia is a common cause of altered mental status in the prehospital setting, justifying the need for obtaining a blood glucose level on any patient who presents as altered. A patient's symptoms as well as the level of blood glucose at which they become symptomatic will vary from patient to patient, likely affected by age, duration of diabetes and treatment regimen. Hypoglycemic patients may exhibit signs of a stroke, drug overdose, traumatic brain injury or mental illness.

Treatment of the hypoglycemic patient with altered mental status or complete unresponsiveness is commonly accomplished with the administration of glucose. Usually, glucose is administered IV for rapid symptom resolution, but is dependent on the ability of the EMS provider to successfully obtain IV access. Glucagon IM is the alternative when IV access is unobtainable. Carstens and Sprehn[14] performed a randomized controlled trial comparing intramuscular glucagon to intravenous glucose with time to symptom resolution as the primary endpoint. Recovery time was significantly quicker in the group that received IV glucose compared to those receiving IM glucagon, with recovery time ranging from 1 to 3 minutes in the glucose group compared to 8 to 21 minutes in the glucagon group. The group receiving IV glucose was noted to have more fluctuation in glucose readings post administration compared to more steady readings in the glucagon group. If IV access can be obtained, glucose remains the preferred treatment, with glucagon being available if an IV is unobtainable.

As with adults, all pediatric patients with an altered mental status need to have their blood glucose checked. Often, the pediatric patient with hypoglycemia is a diagnosed diabetic receiving insulin. As with adults, the pediatric patient should be treated with IV glucose if IV access is attainable or IM glucagon if not.

Studies on most appropriate route for naloxone administration

In hemodynamically stable patients with spontaneous respirations, intranasal naloxone is the preferred route over intramuscular or intravenous given equal efficacy and increased provider safety.

Naloxone (Narcan), commonly used by prehospital care providers as an antidote to opiate overdose, was introduced in 1967.[15] Physiologically, it is a competitive agonist to the mu-opiate receptor, quickly reversing effects of opiates, including altered mental status and respiratory depression. Naloxone can be administered by many routes, including intravenous, intramuscular, subcutaneous, intranasal, endotracheal, sublingual as well as nebulized. Sublingual and oral routes of administration have been found to be less effective than IV or IM.[16, 17] Traditionally, it has been given IV or IM by prehospital care providers due to the rapid and predictable response.[18] However, in 1991, the Occupational Health and Safety Administration mandated implementation of alternative drug delivery systems to decrease exposure to blood-borne pathogens in emergency care providers.[19]

There are two primary issues to consider regarding the use of naloxone for altered mental status by emergency medical services. First, should naloxone be used for every case of altered mental status as part of a "coma cocktail" as initially recommended; and, second, what is the ideal route for giving the drug? As there are no moderate quality recommendations on the safety of empiric use, this will be further discussed in the low quality recommendations section.

Three randomized controlled trials evaluated the most effective route of delivery for naloxone in the prehospital environment. Given that prehospital care providers are at an increased risk of blood-borne exposures due to treating IV drug abusers, there has been great interest in safer non-parenteral routes for pharmacologic treatments such as naloxone to reduce the risk of needlesticks. Naloxone has been found to have almost 100 percent bioavailability through nasal mucosa.[20] Intranasal administration may promote a safer practice environment for paramedics while maintaining effective treatment.

Kerr et al.[21] compared the efficacy of intranasal (IN) to intramuscular (IM) naloxone delivery. Results revealed that there was no significant difference to mean response time or adverse events, although they did find that fewer patients who received intramuscular naloxone were given supplementary doses. Both groups had approximately 25 percent non-responders, similar to reports from other studies.[22, 23] They concluded that given the ease of access and greatly reduced risk of needlestick injury, intranasal naloxone is an effective and safe intervention for initial management of suspected opiate overdose.

Kelly et al.[24] also compared intranasal to intramuscular naloxone in a similarly unblinded, randomized prospective trial. The results indicated that the IM group had a more rapid response than the IN group, but showed no significant difference in the need for additional rescue doses. An unexpected finding was increased rates of agitation after IM naloxone compared to IN naloxone. They concluded that intranasal was effective, although not as effective as the intramuscular route for naloxone. Given the reduced risk of needlestick exposure, they suggest intranasal naloxone be used as first-line therapy in suspected opiate overdose.

The most recent RCT on naloxone by McDermott and Collins[25] compared intranasal (IN) and intravenous (IV) routes. Unlike prior models, this study focused on speed of delivery and satisfaction of advanced paramedics in a classroom-based setting utilizing mannequin models. The authors concluded that the IN route was both faster (by an average of 1.5 minutes) and preferred as safer by participants.

In addition, several prospective cohort and retrospective trials also support the use of intranasal naloxone as the initial treatment for patients with suspected opiate abuse and altered mental status.[26, 22, 23, 27] Other studies[28] have supported the subcutaneous route compared to IV or the use of nebulized naloxone.[29]

Robertson *et al.*[26] found that although time from dose administration to effect was longer in the IN route, time to clinical response from patient contact was not significantly longer when taking into account time to start IV.

Studies on empiric prehospital intubation

Endotracheal intubation is routinely recommended in trauma patients with a GCS below 9 to prevent aspiration of gastric contents and assist with ventilation,[30] although studies have questioned this.[31] There are few prospective studies that examine the ideal GCS in non-trauma patients to indicate a clear need for intubation. Prior studies have found both a large inter-observer variance for the GCS score and that GCS scores correlate poorly with pharyngeal reflexes leading to questions about the validity of GCS as a useful management tool in non-trauma patients.[32, 33] Nielsen et al.[34] studied the need for intubation in unconscious non-trauma patients with a GCS < 9. The majority of patients were not intubated in the prehospital setting except in cases of severe stroke, respiratory failure or cardiac arrest. Only 15 percent of unintubated patients were still unconscious upon arrival to the hospital having either regained consciousness spontaneously or secondary to prehospital treatment. Subsequent intubation of unconscious patients within 24 hours of admission occurred only 19 percent of the time, indicating that unconscious patients may not need intubation prior to hospital arrival except in cases of obvious airway compromise.

Two additional prospective studies evaluated poisoned patients with low GCS score. Donald et al.[35] followed two cohorts of poisoned patients with a GCS < 8 to determine the need for intubation in poisoned patients. One group was intubated and the other followed conservatively with close observation in an intensive environment with physiologic parameters including blood pressure, partial pressure of oxygen and GCS closely monitored. Of the non-intubated group, several required adjunct airway devices, but there was no indication of aspiration pneumonia at discharge and patients had shorter hospital lengths of stay. In a similar study, Duncan and Thakore[36] followed patients with a GCS < 8 with drug or alcohol poisoning in an emergency department observation unit. None of the observed patients had aspiration or required intubation, although a few required admission. Finally, Adnet et al.[37] investigated the association of GCS with difficulty of intubation. Intubation difficulty was reported most frequently in patients with a GCS between 7 and 9 who did not receive sedation and neuromuscular blockade.

Studies on safety of non-transport in diabetic patients with treated hypoglycemia

There have been multiple studies performed to assess the safety of not transporting a patient with insulin-dependent diabetes mellitus (IDDM) to the hospital after successful treatment of hypoglycemia. Successful treatment depends on the return of normal blood sugar levels and the ability of the patient to make an informed decision.[38] Socransky et al.[39] and Mechem et al.[40] both concluded that after administration of glucose and the return of normal mental status, it is safe and efficient to not transport these patients. The rates of relapse within the first 48 hours have not been found to be different in transported versus non-transported patients, with admission to the hospital being rare.[39, 38]

Patients who refuse transportation to the hospital need to be advised of the risk that hypoglycemia may recur. Prehospital providers need to provide education, recommend frequent blood glucose monitoring and suggest follow-up with their primary physicians.

Studies on empiric naloxone administration to all patients with altered mental status

The empiric use of naloxone for all patients with altered mental status was broadly recommended historically, in part due to its lack of adverse effects.[41, 42] Yealy et al.[18] studied the safety of naloxone in the prehospital environment, specifically looking at incidence of vomiting, seizures, hypotension, hypertension and cardiac arrest after its use. The results showed a very low incidence of complications, but also noted only 10.7 percent of patients had any clinical improvement when given naloxone. Safety of naloxone was further prospectively studied by Buajordet et al.,[43] with similar results of low rates of complications. This study advocated continued broad use of naloxone.

Howell and Guly[44] questioned the empiric approach in a study that evaluated whether specific clinical criteria, as opposed to the more broad definition of altered mental status, could more accurately identify patients who would benefit from its use. The study revealed that simply limiting use to altered mental status plus respirations less than 12 per minute would decrease the use of naloxone by 90 percent and still treat 96 percent of positive respondents. Authors note that there is little justification for the use of empiric naloxone in all patients; rather, it should be limited to those with altered mental status and respirations less than 12 per minute.

Summary

In summary, goals of care in patients with altered mental status include focused patient assessment and stabilization of life-threatening causes, including respiratory failure, hypoglycemia and poisoning via opiate overdose. However, the care of these patients in the prehospital care environment remains controversial. In particular, debate exists over prehospital intubation due to unacceptably high rates of failure, even in cases where pharmacologic sedation and neuromuscular blockade are utilized. This is especially true in non-arrest patients, trauma patients and pediatric patients. Multiple studies implore the use of focused assessment to identify patients at high risk of intubation failure and consider the use of basic airway maneuvers such as bag-valve-mask or advanced rescue devices instead of definitive endotracheal intubation. Due to extremely high rates of failure, nasotracheal intubation should never occur in the prehospital environment. Studies also support intubation for signs of obvious airway compromise as opposed to broad recommendations based on Glasgow Coma Scale (GCS). GCS has been shown to correlate poorly with pharyngeal reflexes and does not accurately predict aspiration complications.

Hypoglycemia is a common cause of altered mental status and should be considered in the differential diagnosis. No exact blood glucose level will predict onset or severity of symptoms. Although IV glucose is the treatment of choice, IM glucagon is acceptable when IV access cannot be obtained. Patients with insulin-dependent diabetes mellitus do not need transport if their blood sugar returns to baseline and they have decision-making capacity.

Naloxone is an important medication in patients with suspected opiate overdose as a cause of their altered mental status, as it is both safe and effective. Given the high risk of exposure to blood-borne illnesses via needlestick, most studies advocate the use of needleless delivery routes wherever available, especially intranasal naloxone, which has been studied rigorously. Naloxone does not need to be given to all patients with altered mental status, but can be reserved for those with less than 12 respirations per minute or other reason to suspect opiate overdose.

Key issues for future investigation

The optimal treatment of patients with altered mental status has not been investigated with rigorous scientific trials and there are still many questions to be answered. There continues to be controversy over the efficacy of prehospital endotracheal intubation. Furthermore, given high rates of intubation failure, comparison between definitive airway management and the use of advanced airway adjuvants is long overdue. Additional investigation is also needed to determine if there are selected subgroups of patients that would benefit from prehospital intubation. A large, randomized, controlled trial to evaluate efficacy of endotracheal intubation versus advanced airway equipment or basic maneuvers including bag-valve-mask would ideally be followed by additional studies in selected subpopulations (trauma, pediatrics, etc).

Despite many low-quality studies on limiting naloxone use to patients with suspected opiate abuse, further investigation needs to occur in large, high quality trials using randomization and blinding.

Overall, there is a paucity of data on pediatric patients with altered mental status: although some studies did include all ages, specific questions remain regarding the need for intubation and empiric use of glucose and naloxone.

The following specific questions need to be studied in the prehospital arena for both adults and children:

1. Does intubation of any subgroups of patients with altered mental status improve mortality and morbidity?
2. Are advanced airway adjuncts safe to use in patients with altered mental status regardless of cause?
3. Should blood sugar be assessed prior to empiric treatment with glucose and, if so, what is the cutoff level for treatment?
4. Is empiric naloxone justified solely based on GCS or should only respiratory assessment be used to determine need?
5. Is intranasal naloxone cost-effective in prehospital systems of care?

REFERENCES

1. Durant, E. and Sporer, K. A. (2011). "Characteristics of patients with an abnormal Glasgow Coma Scale score in the prehospital setting," *Western J. Emerg. Med.* 12(1): 30–6.
2. County of San Mateo Health System website (2009). "EMS patient care protocols," available at www.smchealth.org/EMS/Protocols.
3. Wolfson, A. B. (ed.) (2010). *Harwood-Nuss' Clinical Practice of Emergency Medicine* (Philadelphia, PA: Lippincott Williams & Wilkins).
4. Hubble, M. W., Brown, L., Wilfong, D. A. *et al.* (2010). "A meta-analysis of prehospital airway control techniques

part I: orotracheal and nasotracheal intubation success rates," *Prehosp. Emerg. Care* 14(3): 377–401.

5. Spaite, D. W. and Criss, E. A. (2003). "Out-of-hospital rapid sequence intubation: are we helping or hurting our patients?" *Ann. Emerg. Med.* 42(6): 729–30.

6. Gausche, M., Lewis, R. J., Stratton, S. J. *et al.* (2000). "Effect of out-of-hospital pediatric endotracheal intubation on survival and neurological outcome; a controlled clinical trial," *JAMA* 283(6): 783–90.

7. Davis, D. P., Hoyt, D. B., Ochs, M. *et al.* (2003). "The effect of paramedic rapid sequence intubation on outcome in patients with severe traumatic brain injury," *J. Trauma* 54(3): 444–53.

8. Wang, H. E. and Yealy, D. M. (2006). "Out-of-hospital endotracheal intubation: where are we?" *Ann. Emerg. Med.* 47(6): 532–41.

9. Suominen, P., Baillie, C., Kivioja, A. *et al.* (2000). "Intubation and survival in severe paediatric blunt head injury," *Eur. J. Emerg. Med.* 7(1): 3–7.

10. Winchell, R. J. and Hoyt, D. B. (1997). "Endotracheal intubation in the field improves survival in patients with severe head injury. Trauma Research and Education Foundation of San Diego," *Arch. Surg.* 132(6): 592–7.

11. Lecky, F., Bryden, D., Little, R. *et al.* (2008). "Emergency intubation for acutely ill and injured patients," *Cochrane Database Syst. Rev.* (2): CD001429.

12. Lossius, H. M., Roislien, J. and Lockey, D. J. (2012). "Patient safety in pre-hospital emergency tracheal intubation: a comprehensive meta-analysis of the

intubation success rates of EMS providers," *Crit. Care* 16(1): R24.

13. Wang, H. E., Kupas, D. F., Paris, P. M. *et al.* (2003). "Multivariate predictors of failed prehospital endotracheal intubation," *Acad. Emerg. Med.* 10(7): 717–24.

14. Carstens, S. and Sprehn, M. (1998). "Prehospital treatment of severe hypoglycemia: a comparison of intramuscular glucagon and intravenous glucose," *Prehosp. Disaster Med.* 13(2–4): 44–50.

15. Hoffman, J. R., Schriger, D. L., *et al.* (1991). "The empiric use of naloxone in patients with altered mental status: a reappraisal," *Ann. Emerg. Med.* 20(3): 246–52.

16. Maio, R. F., Gaukel, B. and Freeman, B. (1987). "Intralingual naloxone injection for narcotic-induced respiratory depression," *Ann. Emerg. Med.* 16(5): 572–3.

17. Preston, K. L., Bigelow, G. E. and I. A. Liebson. (1990). "Effects of sublingually given naloxone in opioid-dependent human volunteers," *Drug Alcohol Depend.* 25(1): 27–34.

18. Yealy, D. M., Paris, P. M., Kaplan, R. M. *et al.* (1990). "The safety of prehospital naloxone administration by paramedics," *Ann. Emerg. Med.* 19(8): 902–5.

19. Marcus, R., Srivastava, P. U., Bell, D. M. *et al.* (1995). "Occupational blood contact among prehospital providers," *Ann. Emerg. Med.* 25(6): 776–9.

20. Loimer, N., Hofman, P. and Chaundry, H. R. (1994). "Nasal administration of naloxone is as effective as the intravenous route in opiate addicts," *Int. J. Addict.* 29(6): 819–27.

21. Kerr, D., Kelly, A. M., Dietze, P. *et al.* (2009). "Randomized controlled trial comparing the effectiveness and safety of intranasal and intramuscular naloxone for the treatment of suspected heroin overdose," *Addiction* 104(12): 2067–74.

22. Barton, E. D., Colwell, C. B., Wolfe, T. *et al.* (2005). "Efficacy of intranasal naloxone as a needleless alternative for treatment of opioid overdose in the prehospital setting," *J. Emerg. Med.* 29(3): 265–71.

23. Barton, E. D., Ramos, J., Colwell, C. *et al.* (2002). "Intranasal administration of naloxone by paramedics," *Prehosp. Emerg. Care* 6(1): 54–8.

24. Kelly, A. M., Kerr, D., Dietze, P. *et al.* (2005). "Randomised trial of intranasal versus intramuscular naloxone in prehospital treatment for suspected opioid overdose," *Med. J. Aust.* 182(1): 24–7.

25. McDermott, C. and Collins, N. C. (2012). "Prehospital medication administration: a randomised study comparing intranasal and intravenous routes," *Emerg. Med. Int.*, e-pub, Article ID: 476161.

26. Robertson, T. M., Hendey, G. W., Stroh, G. *et al.* (2009). "Intranasal naloxone is a viable alternative to intravenous naloxone for prehospital narcotic overdose," *Prehosp. Emerg. Care* 13(4): 512–15.

27. Merlin, M. A., Saybolt, M., Kapitanyan, R. *et al.* (2010). "Intranasal naloxone delivery is an alternative to intravenous naloxone for opioid overdoses," *Am. J. Emerg. Med.* 28(3): 296–303.

28. Wanger, K., Brough, L., Macmillan, I. *et al.* (1998). "Intravenous vs subcutaneous naloxone for out-of-hospital

management of presumed opioid overdose," *Acad. Emerg. Med.* 5(4): 293–9.

29. Weber, J. M., Tataris, K. L., Hoffman, J. D. *et al.* (2012). "Can nebulized naloxone be used safely and effectively by emergency medical services for suspected opioid overdose?" *Prehosp. Emerg. Care* 16(2): 289–92.

30. American College of Surgeons Committee on Trauma (2012). *Advanced Life Support Course for Physicians* (Chicago, IL: American College of Surgeons).

31. Davis, D. P., Vadeboncoeur, T. F., Ochs, M. *et al.* (2005). "The association between field Glasgow Coma Scale score and outcome in patients undergoing paramedic rapid sequence intubation," *J. Emerg. Med.* 29(4): 391–7.

32. Gill, M. R., Reiley, D. G. and Green, S. M. (2004). "Interrater reliability of Glasgow Coma Scale scores in the emergency department," *Ann. Emerg. Med.* 43(2): 215–23.

33. Moulton, C. and Pennycook, A. G. (1994). "Relation between Glasgow Coma Score and cough reflex," *Lancet* 343(8908): 1261–2.

34. Nielsen, K., Hansen, C. M. and Rasmussen, L. S. (2012). "Airway management in unconscious non-trauma patients," *Emerg. Med. J.* 29(11): 887–9.

35. Donald, C., Duncan, R. and Thakore, S. (2009). "Predictors of the need for rapid sequence intubation in the poisoned patient with reduced Glasgow Coma Score," *Emerg. Med. J.* 26(7): 510–12.

36. Duncan, R. and Thakore, S. (2009). "Decreased Glasgow Coma Scale score does not mandate endotracheal

intubation in the emergency department," *J. Emerg. Med.* 37(4): 451–5.

37. Adnet, F., Borron, S. W., Finot, M. A. *et al.* (1998). "Intubation difficulty in poisoned patients: association with initial Glasgow Coma Scale score," *Acad. Emerg. Med.* 5(2): 123–7.

38. Cain, E., Ackroyd-Stolarz, S., Alexiadis, P. *et al.* (2003). "Prehospital hypoglycemia: the safety of not transporting treated patients," *Prehosp. Emerg. Care* 7(4): 458–65.

39. Socransky, S. J., Pirrallo, R. G., Rubin, J. M. *et al.* (1998). "Out-of-hospital treatment of hypoglycemia: refusal of transport and patient outcome," *Acad. Emerg. Med.* 5(11): 1080–5.

40. Mechem, C. C., Kreshak, A. A., Barger, J. *et al.* (1998). "The short-term outcome of hypoglycemic diabetic patients who refuse ambulance transport after out-of-hospital therapy," *Acad. Emerg. Med.* 5(8): 768–72.

41. Epstein, F. B. and Eilers, M. A. (1988). "Poisoning" in Rosen, P., Baker, F. J., Barkin, R. M. *et al.* (eds). *Emergency Medicine* (St. Louis, MO: C. V. Mosby Co.), p. 330.

42. Rappolt, R. T., Gay, G. R., Decker, W. J. *et al.* (1980). "NAGD regimen for the coma of drug-related overdose," *Ann. Emerg. Med.* 9(7): 357–63.

43. Buajordet, I., Naess, A. C., Jacobsen, D. *et al.* (2004). "Adverse events after naloxone treatment of episodes of suspected acute opioid overdose," *Eur. J. Emerg. Med.* 11(1): 19–23.

44. Howell, M. A. and Guly, H. R. (1997). "A comparison of glucagon and glucose in prehospital hypoglycemia," *J. Accid. Emerg. Med.* 14: 30–2.

INDEX